Keto Diet After 50

How to Stay Healthy With the Ketogenic Diet if You Are Over 50, Including Delicious Recipes to Eat Well Every Day and Lose Weight Fast Without Feeling on a Diet.

Mathilda Schuyler

TABLE OF CONTENTS

INTRODUCTION

Welcome to *Keto Diet After 50,* the book where you will learn all of the information you need to know to begin changing your life! This book will help you harness the keto diet concepts and the science behind it to begin changing your life as you move into your golden years! The Keto diet is a short form for the word "Ketogenic." The Ketogenic diet is a specific diet that involves eating certain foods and eliminating others. This diet is what we will focus on throughout this book.

Before anybody commits to a ketogenic diet, it is important to learn about what it is. Learning the diet details will help you determine whether or not this diet suits your needs and is healthy for your body. Many people with health problems jump into a keto diet without fully understanding what it is, only to create more health problems for themselves.

Before we begin, I want to give a brief disclaimer: This book is not supposed to replace medical advice. It is not responsible for the actions or the results of the reader. Please seek out the advice of a doctor before starting any health program. The author is not a medical doctor, and the information in this book is meant only to supplement your health decisions and actions, not dictate them. Scientists are still researching the wonders of Autophagy at this very moment, even as I write this book. Please enjoy the information provided but also be wise in consuming it.

After reading this book, you will have the tools to decide about the diet you want to follow confidently. I am confident that you will choose the Keto diet and see that this diet is the diet of choice for many people over the age of 50.

CHAPTER 1: INTRODUCTION TO THE KETO DIET

What Is the Keto Diet?

A Ketogenic Diet (or a Keto diet) is a specific diet that involves eating certain foods and eliminating others. This diet came to be because of how it induces a state of Ketosis all of the time in one's body. We will look at what Ketosis is below.

The Keto diet involves eating very high-fat and low-carb (or no carb) foods. You must restrict them to 10% or less of your total daily caloric intake in a Keto diet in terms of carbs. This reduction works out to somewhere around 50 grams of carbohydrates. Protein will contribute about 20 or 30 percent of your daily caloric intake.

What Is Ketosis?

Ketosis is a specific state that the body enters when there is a lack of recently ingested sugars (carbohydrates) or stored sugars; instead, it must use stored fat to get its energy. When the body enters this state, it breaks down its fat stores, and the breakdown of these fat stores creates a specific acid as a by-product. This acid that results is called a *Ketone*. When in a Ketosis state, the brain can use ketones for energy instead of carbohydrates or sugars like it normally would.

This state of Ketosis in the brain induces something called *Autophagy* within the brain cells. Autophagy, as a word, is comprised of two individual parts. Each of these parts on its own is a separate Greek word. The first part of the word is "auto," which means *self,* and the word *"phagy,"* which means *the practice of eating.* Putting these together gives you *"the practice of self-eating,"* which is essentially what Autophagy is. This definition may sound like some type of new-age cannibalism, but it is a very natural process that our cells practice all the time without us being any the wiser. Autophagy is the body's way of cleaning itself out. The process involves small "hunter" particles that go around your body looking for cells or cell components that are old and damaged. The hunter particles then take these cell components apart, getting rid of the damaged parts and saving the useful parts to make new cells later. These hunter cells can also use useful leftover parts to create energy for the body. It is also essential for our bodies' health, as being able to get rid of waste and damaged parts that are no longer useful to us is essential to our health. If we could not get rid of damaged or broken cells, these damaged particles would build up and eventually make us sick. Our bodies are extremely efficient in everything that they do, and waste disposal is no different.

In more recent years, Autophagy's study has been focused more heavily on diet and disease research. These studies are still in their early stages as it has been only a few years shy of sixty years since scientists first discovered Autophagy. Scientists discovered this process in a lab by testing what happened when small organisms went without food for some time. They observed these organisms very closely under a microscope, and they found that their cells had this process of waste disposal and energy creation that was later named Autophagy.

More about Autophagy and its relation to energy production is being studied in recent years, as this topic is interesting to humans. Autophagy can use old cell parts and recycle them to create new energy that the organism (like the human or animal) can use to do its regular functions like walking and breathing. People are now studying what happens when humans rely on this energy production instead of the energy they would get from ingesting food throughout the day. More on this later, though.

Autophagy is said to be the housekeeping function of the body. If you think of your body as your home, Autophagy is the housekeeper you hire to take care of all of the waste and your cells' recycling functions.

One of the housekeeping duties includes removing cell parts that were built wrongly or at the wrong time. Sometimes cells make mistakes, and these mistakes can lead to the creation of proteins or other cell parts in error. When this happens, we need something within the cell to get rid of these errors so that they do not take up space or get in the way of other processes within the cell. Further, sometimes useful parts of the cell will become damaged somehow, and they will need to get removed to make way for a new part to take its place. These cell parts can include those that create DNA or those that create the proteins needed to make the DNA.

Another duty of Autophagy is to protect the body from disease and pathogens. Pathogens are bacteria or viruses that can infect our cells and our bodies if they do not properly defend against them. Autophagy works to kill the cells within our body infected by these pathogens to get rid of them before they can spread. In this way, Autophagy plays a part in our immune system as it acts as a supplement to our immune cells whose sole function is to protect us from invasions by disease and infection.

Autophagy also functions to help the body's cells regulate themselves when there are stressors placed upon them. These stressors can be things like a lack of food for the cell or physical stresses placed on the cell. This regulation helps maintain a standard cell environment despite factors that can change like food availability. Autophagy can do things like break down cell parts for food to provide the cell with nutrients.

It was discovered that Autophagy happens in all organisms that are multi-cellular, like animals and plants, in addition to humans. These larger organisms and how Autophagy works in their cells are less well-understood. Scientists are now conducting more studies on humans and how diet changes can affect their body's Autophagy.

The other function that Autophagy serves is that it helps cells to carry out their death when it is time for them to die. There are times when cells get programmed to die because of several different factors. Sometimes these cells need assistance in their death, and Autophagy can help them with this or clean up after their death. The human body is all about life and death, and these processes are continually going on without our knowledge to keep us healthy and in good form.

The state of Autophagy in the brain boasts many benefits for the brain cells. This process works because the Ketones in the brain induce Autophagy by signaling to the brain cells that there are low energy sources, so the brain is using ketones for energy. If you remember, low energy levels are a signal for Autophagy. It is not completely understood much further than this, but Ketosis and its induction of Autophagy have produced many positive effects for the brain, like brain cells' protection. This benefit leads to a reduction in the likelihood of diseases like Alzheimer's or Parkinson's.

Autophagy is a process that happens within the body that has been going on since the beginning of humans. It is only recently that people began harnessing this process to achieve desired positive results. These positive results have led people to control their bodies' environment by turning to the Keto diet. The Keto diet allows people to reach a state of Ketosis and Autophagy, which leads to numerous benefits, which we will learn about in the next chapter.

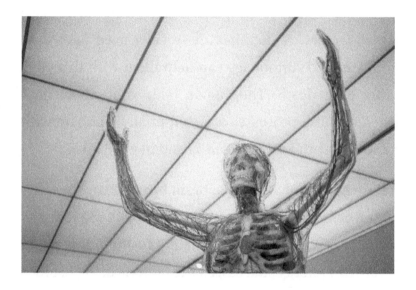

What Does Ketosis Look and Feel Like? (How to Tell if Your Body Is in Ketosis)

The ketones produced from the breakdown of fat stores get released in urine, and this is how you can tell when your body is in a state of Ketosis. It is beneficial to know when you are in this state if you are attempting to get your body to break down fat stores, knowing that this is the state you are in, you then know that your methods are functioning. If you are interested, you can test this using test strips, which will tell you your urine's acidity—the more acidic your urine, the higher presence of ketones.

Who Should Follow the Keto Diet?

- Those pursuing weight loss
- Those looking to improve their health
- Those looking to reduce inflammation
- Those looking to manage an inflammatory disease or condition

You still may want to consult a doctor for those in generally good health before deciding to begin any dieting plan. It will prove extremely beneficial to explore the pros and cons of a diet plan with a healthcare professional before making an informed decision for yourself. If you decide that you would like to try it, there is no harm in keeping your doctor updated now and then so that they can monitor your health. Keeping them updated can also be beneficial because they can tell you if you are making progress of any sort and give you their recommendations along the way. Your doctor can also monitor you to ensure that no complications will result from your diet plan choice.

Things to Keep In Mind for People Over the Age of 50

Depending on your age, you must ensure that you approach the diet with a certain safety level. The elderly are at a vulnerable age, as people of an older age are more susceptible to diseases and illnesses of any sort. They also tend to be smaller in size and have less body fat than they did when they were younger.

For these reasons, Physicians strongly advise people in the elderly age category to use precaution when choosing the keto diet as a form of weight loss and health improvement. This population needs all of the nutrients that they can receive from the foods they eat and the regular blood sugar levels that regularly ingest food throughout the day. As they do not have as much fat stored on their bodies, often they do not have the fat stores needed to break down fat for energy while cutting out carbohydrates. Thus, fasting can be dangerous for the elderly, and they should only follow this kind of diet plan with the help and guidance of a doctor.

CHAPTER 2: BENEFITS OF THE KETO DIET

There are numerous benefits that our bodies can gain from eating according to the keto diet. Many of these benefits come from the fact that Ketosis leads to Autophagy, as you now know. The simplest and most basic way to tell that it is a benefit to our bodies is that our bodies have preserved it for this long. As I mentioned earlier in this book, our bodies are extremely efficient and are designed for survival. If something that does not contribute to our survival or our health, our body will usually get rid of it or lower its functioning as it can use its resources elsewhere for more benefit. Autophagy is still functioning well, and many positive things come of it, which is why it is still an important cell function in multi-cellular beings to this day. We will look at more of the benefits below.

Benefits of the Keto Diet

The Keto diet comes with several benefits, some of which we have seen in this book's first chapter. Here, we will examine the benefits in a little more detail.

1. *Skin Health*

As you likely know, skin health can be closely related to diet and sugar intake. Since the Keto diet reduces carbohydrates and sugars, it can lead to decreased acne levels and improved overall skin health. This improvement is because ingesting high sugar levels leads to dramatic rises and dips in blood sugar levels, which affects a person's skin health.

2. *Weight Loss*

Metabolism is a large term that describes the breakdown of one thing to create energy. It is all of the body's processes that work together to maintain life in more specific terms. This benefit happens when you eat food, and it is broken down to create energy for your body to function. This energy creation also happens on a smaller level in each cell of your body by Autophagy. Autophagy carries cell components to the lysosome, and the breakdown of these cell components is used to create energy for the cell. As we learned earlier, Autophagy is initiated by low nutrition levels in the cell, and thus it creates energy for that cell. In this way, it contributes to the body's overall metabolism by creating energy by breaking something down.

When cells are experiencing a lack of nutrition and Autophagy is triggered, the body releases hormones to use the energy it is creating in the most efficient way possible. These hormones make the fat stores more easily broken down and more accessible as a source of energy. Because of this, the body's rate of metabolism increases during these times of cellular starvation.

This process leads to weight loss because it causes the body to break down its fat stores. This breakdown is beneficial for a person's health in general, but it is also beneficial for their weight loss.

3. Autophagy and Brain Health

As I briefly mentioned in the previous chapter, the Keto diet is very beneficial for a person's brain cells. This benefit is because of something called Autophagy that we learned about earlier.

As a reminder, Autophagy is a process that the body uses to clean itself out. This process involves small "hunter" particles that go around your body's cells, looking for cell components that are old and damaged. The hunter particles then take these cell components apart, getting rid of the damaged parts and saving the useful parts to make new cells later. These hunter cells can also use useful leftover parts to create energy for the body.

The benefits of this process are far-reaching. This process leads to a clean and efficient environment within your body's cells and keeps everything functioning well. It also reduces the risk of diseases like cancer.

Dementia is a blanket term for a combination of symptoms of cognitive declines, such as forgetfulness and disorientation. Alzheimer's disease is one common example of dementia. One cause of dementia is cell death, which we know by now involves Autophagy. This brain cell death happens over some time and includes gradual cognitive decline as this happens. The actual causes of dementia, including Alzheimer's, are not well known, but what is known is that this steady decline is linked to abnormal cell death.

When you are eating according to the Keto diet, Ketosis's state caused acts as a signal for Autophagy in the brain. Autophagy in the brain cleans the brain cells and keeps them healthy. This process reduces your risk of cancers in the brain or diseases of the brain like Alzheimer's. Eating according to a Keto diet is not only beneficial for the body, as we will see, but it is also beneficial for the mind. Aside from preventing disease, it helps to keep your brain sharp and functioning well. We will look at this in more detail soon.

Health Benefits That You Can Expect

1. Cancer Prevention

We previously discussed how the Keto diet could lead to a decreased risk of brain cancer, but it can also reduce your risk of other cancers. We discussed that Autophagy cleans out the body's cells; it does this in other parts of the body and not just in the brain. When it does this, it can clean out cells that could become cancerous or cells that are already cancerous, preventing many different types of cancer. It has also been shown to be an effective cancer treatment, along with chemotherapy and radiation. Further, the stabilizing effects that this diet has on blood sugar levels can also reduce the risk of some cancers that have been associated with blood sugar regulation complications.

2. *Improved Heart Health*

If the Keto diet consists of healthy fats and fats from animal sources (we will look at this more later), it can lead to better heart health. This benefit is because it can reduce cholesterol levels.

3. *Seizure Reduction*

In people who suffer from epilepsy, ketones' presence during Ketosis resulting from the Keto diet can reduce seizures. This benefit is effective in children suffering from this disease.

4. *Polycystic Ovarian Syndrome (PCOS) Management*

PCOS or Polycystic Ovarian Syndrome is something that many women suffer from. This disease leads women's ovaries to develop cysts, leading to very painful periods, weight gain, and infertility. It has been shown that a diet high in carbohydrates can negatively affect this disease and exacerbate symptoms. Following the Keto diet showed an improvement in women's general health with PCOS, reduced their symptoms (including leading to weight loss) and helped mitigate the disease's progression.

5. *Immune System Strengthening*

Autophagy is important for our immune system function. As I briefly mentioned in the previous chapter, Autophagy plays a part in the immune system by killing infected cells before spreading and infecting other cells. This function of Autophagy has perhaps developed over time to adapt to the changes in pathogens that humans are exposed to these days, and it has become quite a benefit to us.

The way that Autophagy assists the immune system is similar to how it carries pathogens to the lysosomes to be broken down. When there is a pathogen present, an autophagosome will be created within the cell in just the same way that it is created when there are cell debris and a low level of nutrients. This pathogen will be engulfed by the autophagosome and carried to the lysosome. This type of Autophagy is not for recycling and energy production, but breakdown and destruction. By this process, which is very similar to energy production, the cell can be rid of pathogens that infected it without the need for a full-blown immune response. This response, of course, depends on the level of infection in the body. This process that is already occurring in our cells expands its function to serve another purpose, which turns out to be greatly beneficial for our general health.

6. *Inflammation Reduction And Management*

Inflammation is a reaction that occurs in the body in response to things such as pathogens or irritations. Inflammation is a response intended to protect us from whatever signaled the inflammation to occur. It does this by increasing the number of inflammatory cells in the area where the irritant or pathogen is located. The inflammatory cells remove the irritant, promote new cell growth to replace cells damaged by the irritant, and promote overall repair of the area.

Autophagy plays a large role in inflammation as it has a big effect on the inflammatory cells involved. Autophagy can keep inflammatory cells alive by breaking down old and damaged cell parts and keeping the cells healthy and in good working order. It does this in the same way that it keeps any of our other cells working and alive. These inflammatory cells are necessary to keep the organism itself healthy by reaching the damage or disease site and clearing it out. These inflammatory cells have many jobs to do, and they must stay healthy. Autophagy ensures this and thus has a big impact on the overall health of the organism.

On the outside of the body, inflammation can be identified by redness, swelling, heat to the touch, and pain. This inflammation can happen when there is an infection, a physical injury, or any other assault to that area. Inflammation may seem like it is an annoying problem that your body causes you. Still, it is a sign of your body working tirelessly to keep you healthy and remove whatever isn't supposed to be there, making you sick. We would not be able to heal if it were not for inflammation and Autophagy's role in inflammation. Autophagy also plays a role in reducing inflammation, especially in the brain. Since Autophagy can both keep cells alive and to cause their death, it can control the presence of inflammatory cells and control their exit when the irritant has been removed. By inducing Autophagy in your body, you can reduce inflammation by having the inflammatory cells be broken down and removed.

- *Acute Inflammation*

There are different types of inflammation. The first one we will discuss is the one you are likely most familiar with, acute inflammation. Acute inflammation has a rapid onset but usually only lasts until the bacteria or the injury is gone. Examples of this include a cut or scrape, tonsillitis, sinusitis, and bronchitis. The inflammatory response occurs at the first sign of infection or virus in the body. These inflammatory cells are no longer present after they have successfully gotten rid of the problem in that area of the body.

- *Chronic Inflammation*

The other type of inflammation is chronic inflammation. Chronic inflammation occurs over a long period, from months to years, and has a slower onset than acute inflammation. Acute inflammation can become chronic inflammation if the infection or the injury is not resolved from the initial inflammatory immune response. Chronic inflammation can also occur because of consistent exposure over a long period to a low level of irritants like allergens or chemicals. When inflammation becomes chronic, we begin to see diseases develop.

Inflammation is beneficial and necessary for proper healing and maintenance of good health. Still, when it occurs over a long period (such as years), this lasting inflammation can create problems in the body.

Inflammatory Diseases

"Inflammatory Disease" is an umbrella term for various diseases that involve inflammation in some parts of the body, usually over a long period. Examples of these diseases include the following;

- *Allergies*

Allergies to something like a cat when you visit someone's house can come about quickly when in the cat's presence and be gone after a few days once the irritant is removed. Sometimes, however, the inflammation caused by allergies can become chronic and lead to a condition like hay fever. This chronic condition happens when the nasal pathways become inflamed to protect the person from inhaling any more of the irritant (like pollen or grass); however, this inflammation can become quite irritating to the person after a few weeks of experiencing it. They will experience things like a stuffed nose, making it difficult for the person to go about their regular lives. At this point, inflammation that is supposed to help the person becomes more of a burden.

- *Asthma*

Asthma is a disease caused by inflammation of the tubes that connect and move air to and from the lungs, as well as the tubes within the lungs. Because these airways are inflamed, they are extra sensitive to everything that the lungs inhale, especially irritants of any sort. When an irritant is inhaled, the already inflamed airways become even more swollen, making it very difficult for the person to breathe. Asthma and allergies are closely linked and can act in similar ways or tandem in the body. Like allergies, chronic inflammation can be caused by environmental factors such as pollution in the air or chronic mold exposure.

- *Inflammatory Bowel Disease*

Inflammatory bowel disease is another disease caused by chronic inflammation. Within the term, Inflammatory bowel disease (IBD), several more specific conditions are characterized by the digestive tract's inflammation. IBD is caused by an abnormal response in the gut to certain foods, or bacteria and viruses, leading to chronic inflammation.

There are many symptoms that the digestive tract's inflammation can cause, including nausea, lack of appetite, fever, fatigue, and abnormal stools.

One example of an IBD is Crohn's Disease, where any part of the digestive tract can be the site of inflammation. The food that a person puts in their body is very important when they have IBD, as the food will have to go through the digestive tract, and thus the inflamed areas will be involved every time the person ingests food.

All of these inflammatory diseases can come about but can also be improved by the presence of Autophagy. Autophagy can keep this inflammation alive, but it can also remedy and reduce these diseases' occurrence if induced at the right times. We will look at this further in the next chapter.

- *Obesity*

While there are many causes of obesity, one of the more recently discovered causes may be related to Autophagy or, rather, dysfunction of Autophagy within the body. This result is because of the way the metabolism is affected. As Autophagy becomes improperly regulated, it can lead to various metabolic disorders, obesity being one of them. This obesity can be caused by problems related to autophagy function in fat tissues, especially leading to problems in the breakdown of fat tissues.

How It Will Benefit People Over 50 Specifically

There are benefits to the keto diet that prove to be more beneficial for those over the age of 50. As you age, there are certain things to keep in mind regarding your health and the health benefits you should be seeking when choosing a diet plan.

1. *Longevity*

The state of Ketosis and Autophagy is more important than we may even realize as it plays a large role in the survival of the living organisms it acts within. It does this by being especially sensitive to the levels of nutrients and energy within a cell. When the nutrient levels lower, Autophagy breaks down cell parts, creating nutrients and energy for the cell. If it weren't for this process, the cells would not maintain their ideal functioning environment. They may begin to make more mistakes and even lower their functioning abilities altogether. So much goes on inside a cell that they need to work effectively at all times. Autophagy makes this possible, which is what makes it such an essential function.

Autophagy is essential for the longevity of the organism. Autophagy has been shown to affect aging, so it plays such a large role in longevity. The reason for this is twofold. The first reason is that the cells that it acts in are often damaged or injured. By way of Autophagy, the disease or virus that is attempting to infect the organism is unable to spread, allowing the organism to continue living a relatively healthy life. This type of disease control increases the longevity of the organism.

The second reason is that Autophagy is essential to maintaining the health of specific tissues and organs, which keeps them running smoothly and functioning at their best, which is another factor that influences lifespan. If the organs and tissues are healthy, the organism will be healthy and will keep living.

In these two ways, Autophagy plays a large role in the organisms' longevity and lifespan and their cells.

2. General Quality Of Life

While at first, Autophagy may seem like it has nothing to do with its quality, it has many indirect effects on quality of life in general. As you will see in this chapter, Autophagy can affect the body in many positive and negative ways. Autophagy can cause diseases, and it can also prevent them. It can maintain and create the organism's health and the possibility to also create and maintain disease within the body. Everything in the body comes down to what happens at a cellular level, as it works in a bottom-up way. Whatever happens at the cellular level will work its way up, affecting everything at the larger levels before eventually affecting the body as a whole. We will become aware of what is happening at a cellular level once its effects work their way up to our consciousness.

Having a disease, especially one that involves inflammation of some part of the body, can cause high levels of pain and discomfort daily for the person affected. This pain and discomfort affect the quality of life as the person living with pain must take this with them in everything they do.

On the other hand, Autophagy can affect a person's quality of life by maintaining their health and eliminating it. Inflammation in the short term helps to get rid of diseases, bacterial infections, and any sort of injury. By effectively eliminating disease and injury promptly, the person's quality of life is greatly increased as their health is improved.

When it comes to the quality of life, Autophagy has been shown to benefit mental health. Intermittent fasting, which induces Autophagy, has decreased instances of depression and food-related disorders such as binge eating. Its benefits for weight loss also improve body image, confidence, and overall self-satisfaction in adults who practice it for one month or more.

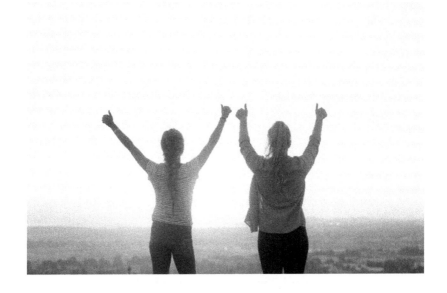

Precautions to Take Regarding the Keto Diet

There are some things to keep in mind when fasting or when changing to a new diet. When it comes to the kept diet or a low-carb diet specifically, there is something known as the

"Keto Flu" you may experience. This type of flu comes with a list of symptoms caused by the body trying to adapt to a diet with a dramatic reduction in carbohydrates. These symptoms include nausea, fatigue, headaches, constipation, and intense sugar cravings.

These symptoms could begin somewhere in the first day or two, and the amount of time they last can vary from a week to multiple weeks. If you experience this, you can take steps to stay healthy and help your body adapt to this dramatic change in diet.

1. The first step is to ensure you are drinking enough liquids, including water and electrolytes. However, the one thing to keep in mind is that some electrolyte beverages contain a lot of sugar, so beware of their carbohydrate content and try to choose one that is not very sugary. As I mentioned previously, some dehydration often comes with the keto diet or a restricting diet of any sort, so ensure that you are adequately replacing these fluids lost. About two liters should be a good amount.

2. Increasing your salt intake can also help with the keto flu. When you restrict your carbohydrate intake, you will lose salt through your urine, so replacing this is

also important. Contrary to what you may have heard, sometimes it is necessary to ingest salt, especially if you don't have an overly salty diet.

3. To achieve both points 1 and 2, you can drink broth to increase salt and liquid levels.

4. If you feel cramps due to dehydration, eating foods like bananas or tomatoes will help with the muscle cramps.

5. When you adapt to the initial period of the keto diet, you will need to scale back your exercise level for the first week. You will want to exercise to a much lighter level at first and gradually increase your exercise level as you adapt more and more.

Who Should Not Follow the Keto Diet?

Some populations may experience complications when following a strict diet because of certain health risks it may pose. While the keto diet can provide countless health benefits, the following groups of people should consult a medical professional before beginning the diet.

- *Those who have Kidney problems*

People suffering from kidney disease need more calories than people who are in good health. They need the nutrition that these calories provide them with as well. For this reason, those with kidney problems such as kidney stones, kidney failure, or any other disease of the kidneys should consult a doctor before severely limiting their carbohydrate intake.

- *Those who have Liver problems*

Dieting can be hard on the liver, as it is the liver that makes the ketones that the body uses for energy while using fat instead of carbohydrates for energy. When carbohydrates are not available, the liver works overtime. While this can provide many benefits, it may not be safe for those who have liver diseases. If a person's liver is already stressed because of their disease, it is not good to stress the liver by cutting out carbohydrates.

- *Women who are trying to conceive*

When women are trying to conceive, their bodies are sensitive to the state of the body's internal environment. This sensitivity is because the body will not allow conception if the environment is not ideal for a healthy fetus's growth. It is important to ensure that your body is in good shape and has enough nutrients if you are trying to conceive so that the body is confident that it will be able to grow a healthy baby.

- *Those who are underweight*

If you are underweight, your body will not have access to the fat stores that it would turn to when cutting out carbohydrates and using fat stores for energy. In this case, fasting can be dangerous because without these fat stores to break down and use up as energy, the body can severely lack energy and nutrients.

- *Those who are pregnant*

When pregnant, your body is attempting to grow a healthy baby. The baby cannot go without the proper nutrients and food that it needs to grow to do this. Everything that you ingest while pregnant will be shared with your baby through the umbilical cord. If you do not have enough nutrients, the development of the baby could suffer.

- *Those who are breastfeeding*

While breastfeeding, nutrients and minerals from everything, the mother ingests are passed to the baby through the milk. Some studies show that breast milk's taste can change depending on what the mother has most recently ingested. For this reason, it is important that the mother remains nourished and fed so that the baby is getting proper nourishment as well. The first few months, while the mother is breastfeeding, are essential to the baby's development, and breast milk is the main reason. Keeping the breast milk full of nutrients is essential. For this reason, avoiding carbohydrates is not something that a person should do when breastfeeding.

- *Women who have irregular periods*

It has been shown that dieting or restricting carbohydrates can cause women to have irregular periods due to the hormone production and secretion changes that it can cause. Those who experience this already should avoid fasting without consulting a doctor first.

- *Those with a history of eating disorders*

For people who have a history of eating disorders of any sort, diets can be quite tricky. These people need to be careful when restricting or controlling food intake in any way. Food-related planning and restricting can act as a trigger for those who have a history of eating disorders. It is not recommended that those people participate in dieting of any sort. Further, you should consult a doctor if you are considering the keto diet.

- *Those who are below the age of eighteen*

For people in their teen years, or especially children, dieting or restricting food intake is not a necessary tool for weight loss or health improvement. Any diet is not advisable for this population as they are still growing and developing and need all of the nutrients that they ingest. They also tend to be more active, and because of this, they likely use up more than the number of calories they eat daily. At these ages, the body needs the calories that come from carbohydrates to grow and change in the proper ways to prepare it for adulthood.

- *Those who have conditions of the heart*

Those with conditions of the heart should take extra care if they are dieting. This precaution is necessary because their medication schedule is very rigid, and it must be taken with food. As this is not a medication schedule that can be adjusted, changing their diet without first consulting a doctor is not a good idea for patients with this medication schedule. Further, some heart patients experience shortness of breath or lightheadedness, and changing carbohydrate intake can exacerbate these symptoms if blood sugar becomes low.

As there are many different heart conditions, it is necessary to consult a physician before deciding if dieting is right for you.

- *Those with diabetes*

Because people with diabetes have struggled with their blood sugar, dieting is likely not a good choice for them unless instructed by a doctor. When you restrict carbohydrates, your body must find other sources of sugar to maintain blood sugar. In people with diabetes, this can cause complications for their already sensitive blood sugar levels.

For people with diabetes, having their blood sugar reach levels too high or too low can be very dangerous as their body has a hard time regulating it. Following the keto diet may pose serious health risks for this population.

The goal is to improve your health, so ensuring that you are doing so in a healthy way is key.

CHAPTER 3: FOODS TO EAT ON THE KETO DIET

In this chapter, we will begin learning about the specific foods that are a part of the Keto diet. This chapter will give you an idea of what you can expect to eat when you begin following this diet. I will begin by reviewing what the Keto diet includes and what it restricts, as discussed in the first chapter of this book. Remember that the Keto diet involves eating very high-fat and low-carb (or no carb) foods.

When following a keto diet, the following are true;

- Carbohydrates are restricted to 10% or less of your total daily caloric intake. This restriction works out to somewhere around 50 grams of carbohydrates.
- Protein will contribute about 20 or 30 percent of your daily caloric intake.
- Fats are included in this diet intentionally.

When it comes to fats, there are different types. Many people refer to them as "good" and "bad" fats. But we will instead call them healthy fats and unhealthy fats. Most of the time, when you think of fats, you likely think of fried foods and packaged baked goods. There are many other foods, however, that contain healthy types of fats.

This particular diet works by eliminating the carbohydrates you would normally eat to give you energy throughout the day so that your body has to turn to other energy sources. This lack of carbohydrates puts your body in a state of Ketosis (hence the name), as you now know.

Best Foods to Eat On the Keto Diet

You may be wondering what types of foods you can eat on a keto diet. As a reminder, in general, the Ketogenic diet involves eating very high-fat and low-carb (or no carb) foods. In terms of carbs, they are restricted to 10% or less of your total daily caloric intake in a Keto diet. This amount works out to somewhere around 50 grams of carbohydrates. Protein will contribute about 20 or 30 percent of your daily caloric intake. We will look at some examples of the foods included in a Ketogenic diet in this section.

Some healthy fats are essential components of any person's diet, as our bodies cannot make the beneficial compounds that they contain; thus, we rely solely on our diet to get them. These compounds are Omega-3 Fatty Acids, monounsaturated and polyunsaturated fats. Below are some healthy sources of these compounds;

- Avocados
- Healthy, plant-based oils including olive oil and canola oil

- Hemp, chia, and flax seeds
- Walnuts

Fish is a great way to get healthy fats when following a Keto diet. Certain fish are very low in carbohydrates but high in good fats, making them perfect for this diet. They also contain minerals and vitamins that will be good for your health. Salmon is a great fish to eat on this diet as it is essentially carbohydrate-free. Many fish also include essential fatty acids that we can only get through our diet. Other fish that are good to eat on a Keto diet are;

- Sardines
- Mackerel
- Herring
- Trout
- Albacore Tuna

Shellfish are also a good choice, though some contain small amounts of carbohydrates, so it is important to keep this in mind when including them in a Keto diet. The following shellfish are arranged in order of increasing carbohydrate content. They range from 3 grams to 7 grams of carbohydrates per 100-gram serving.

- Squid
- Oysters

- Octopus
- Clams
- Mussels

Vegetables are included in a Keto diet, as they contain low numbers of calories and carbohydrates but have many beneficial vitamins and minerals. The body does not digest fiber, so it is good to eat vegetables containing fiber as they help you feel full without actually filling your body with digestible carbohydrates. When looking at which vegetables to eat, take the total amount of carbohydrates and subtract from it the amount of fiber to determine how many carbs your body will absorb from it. Some examples of fibrous vegetables include the following;

- Celery
- Spinach
- Brussels Sprouts
- Asparagus
- Bok Choy
- Cabbage
- Green Beans
- Artichokes

Some vegetables, however, include high amounts of carbohydrates. These vegetables include starchy vegetables such as root vegetables. You must be careful when including these vegetables in a Keto diet since they are not too high in fiber but contain a high starch content.

- Potatoes
- Beets
- Yams
- Squash

Cheese may surprise you as a good choice in a diet plan, but it is great for the Ketogenic diet as it contains high-fat content but very low carb content, which is true for all types of cheese. Cheese has also been shown to protect against heart disease in some studies and help with fat loss and body composition improvements.

- Cheddar cheese
- Ricotta cheese
- Swiss cheese
- Parmigiano Reggiano
- Feta cheese

Avocados are a great option for healthy fat for anyone, especially those on a Ketogenic diet. Avocados are high in fiber, so their carbohydrate content is reduced to only about two grams of carbohydrates per 100-gram serving. They are high in healthy fats at the same time, so they are the ideal Keto food. They also contain vitamins and minerals that are healthy for improved overall health. Avocados have been shown to reduce "bad" cholesterol and improve "good" cholesterol.

Meat and Poultry make up a large part of a Ketogenic diet. Meats and Poultry that are fresh and not processed do not include any carbohydrates but contain high protein levels. Eating lean meats when on a low-carbohydrate diet helps to maintain your strength and muscle mass that could otherwise decrease due to decreased carbohydrate intake. Grass-fed meats, in particular, are rich in antioxidants and beneficial fats, which is great for a Ketogenic diet.

Eggs are another amazing Ketogenic food. They have virtually no carbohydrates and contain protein. Eggs help you feel full for longer and keep blood sugar levels consistent, which is great for overall health. The whole egg is good for you, as the yolk is where the nutrients are. The cholesterol found within egg yolks has also been shown to reduce heart disease risk, despite what most people think. When on a Keto diet, do not be afraid of the yolk of the egg.

There are numerous oils that you can find on the shelves of any grocery store. Knowing which to choose can be difficult. In this section, we will look at the best oils for a Ketogenic diet. The following oils are known to be good sources of healthy fats;

- *Coconut Oil*

This oil is extremely versatile and can be used in cooking, skincare, coffee, etc. Coconut oil specifically has been shown to increase Ketosis in the brain. Coconut oil can also lead to prolonged states of Ketosis, which extends the benefits over the longer-term.

- *Olive oil*

Olive oil is great for reducing inflammation, and it is carbohydrate-free.

Just as olive oil is good for the Keto diet, so are **olives.** They have the same benefits of olive oil, but in solid form instead. Since you would not enjoy drinking olive oil, eating olives is a great way to get these benefits in a quick, snack form.

Greek Yogurt is a food that is high in protein but small amounts of carbohydrates. **Cottage Cheese** is another similar food that contains high protein and low carbohydrates. They both help you feel full from eating small amounts and keeping you full for longer because of the protein they contain, which keeps giving you energy for a prolonged period. These can be put together with other foods or eaten alone.

Nuts and **Seeds** are foods that are high in fat and fiber and low in carbohydrates. The carbohydrate count varies among nuts and seeds, but those with the lowest carbohydrates are below. All of the following include between 0 and 3 grams of carbohydrates;

- Brazil Nuts
- Pecans
- Walnuts
- Flaxseeds
- Chia Seeds
- Macadamia nuts
- Sesame seeds
- Almonds

Berries are different from other fruits in that they are low in carbohydrates. Most fruits are high in carbohydrates because of the sugars they contain, but berries are an exception. They are high in fiber and very low in carbohydrates. In particular, **raspberries** and **blackberries** have the same amount of digestible carbohydrates as fiber, making them very healthy. Berries also contain many healthy antioxidants and anti-inflammatory compounds. Other berries include **blueberries** and **strawberries.**

Butter is a food that is high in fat but low in carbohydrates (virtually zero). This small amount of carbohydrates is also true for **cream.** Cream and butter have been shown to promote fat loss and reduce stroke and heart attack risk.

Coffee and **tea** are fine to consume on a Keto diet, but they must be unsweetened. These drinks on their own contain no calories or carbohydrates, but they are healthy because of their antioxidants and their influence on the body's metabolism. Teas like green tea and black tea are especially good for the body's metabolism. It is fine to add cream to coffee or tea on the Ketogenic diet, but only cream and not low-fat milk as it contains sugar.

Cocoa is a superfood, which is why it is included in this list. Cocoa and dark chocolate are rich in nutrients like antioxidants and have been shown to reduce the risk of high blood pressure, heart disease, and stroke. When choosing a bar of dark chocolate, it is important to pick one unsweetened and no less than 70% cocoa so that there are not too many carbohydrates contained within.

Legumes are a great source of protein and fiber, and there are many different types to choose from. These include the following;

- All sorts of beans, including black beans, green beans, and kidney beans
- Peas
- Lentils of all colors
- Chickpeas
- Peas

Seeds are another great source of nutrients, vitamins, and minerals, and they are very versatile. These include the following;

- Sesame seeds
- Pumpkin seeds
- Sunflower seeds
- Hemp, flax, and chia seeds are all especially good for your health.

Nuts are a great way to get protein if you choose not to eat meat or vegan. They also are packed with nutrients. Some examples are below.

- Almonds
- Brazil Nuts

- Cashews
- Macadamia nuts
- Pistachios
- Pecans

In a Ketogenic diet, it is important to choose the carbohydrates you will include wisely, as there is not much room to include them. Choose food sources that are not very carbohydrate-dense and that include other beneficial nutrients. Some people on a keto diet also choose to supplement Ketones, which can help get your body into a state of Ketosis quicker and help you feel the benefits of the mental sharpness you need.

When it comes to carbohydrates, these should be consumed in **whole grains**, as they are high in fiber, which will help prevent overeating. Whole grains also include essential minerals- those that we can only get from our diet, just like those essential compounds found in healthy fats. These essential minerals are selenium, magnesium, and copper. Sources of these whole grains include the following;

- Quinoa
- Rye, Barley, buckwheat
- Whole grain oats
- Brown rice

- Whole grain bread can be hard to find these days in the grocery store, as many brown loaves of bread disguise themselves as whole grain when, in fact, they are not. However, there are whole grain loaves of bread if you take the time to look at the ingredients list.

Raw Food Vs. Cooked Food

We will now discuss something that is heavily debated within the diet and nutrition world. Raw versus cooked food. Some people are strongly committed to the idea that raw food is better for your diet than cooked food. Raw food includes food that is unprocessed, unheated, uncooked, and fermented.

Benefits of a Raw Diet

People of these beliefs believe the following points;

1. *Vitamins*

When you cook your food, some of the nutrients that the food contained when it was raw may not be present anymore when cooked. Specifically, this can happen with several vitamins. This removal of vitamins is because some vitamins are water-soluble, meaning that they dissolve in water, so if you are boiling a vegetable, the vitamins from the food may dissolve in the water exit the food itself. Water-soluble vitamins include vitamin C and the B vitamins. The majority of the vitamins that are lost during cooking will be water-soluble. Still, some others like Vitamin A and some other minerals may also become deactivated through cooking, but to a much lesser degree. Since boiling vegetables can cause them to lose vitamins, a possible solution could be to cook them differently, such as roasting, steaming, or frying them. This different cooking method will lead to less vitamin loss as these methods use much less water. Another possible solution could be boiling a vegetable for less time, resulting in less nutrient loss.

2. *Enzymes*

The other thing that raw foodists (those who consume a raw diet) believe is that many enzymes within the food are denatured during the cooking process because of the heat. These enzymes can aid your gut's digestion processes, but it will require more enzyme recruitment within your gut to break down the food if they are denatured. Raw foodists believe that this ends up putting long-term stress on your digestive system. While it is true that enzymes become denatured at high heat levels, there is little scientific evidence that this causes any undue stress on the body.

3. *Toxicity*

Some extreme raw foodists believe that a cooked food diet is unhealthy and toxic for the human body.

Drawbacks of a Raw Diet

On the other hand, though, some drawbacks are worth noting when considering a raw food diet.

1. *Vitamins*

While it is true that some vitamins are destroyed during the cooking process of food, there are others, however, that are more readily available for your body to use when your food is cooked.

2. *Challenging*

It is quite difficult to follow a complete or even 70% raw food diet. A person will rarely be able to stick to a raw diet on a long-term basis.

3. *Bacteria and Illness*

When it comes to raw foods, some can be dangerous to consume. Some bacteria are present in foods that are killed during the cooking process, which is why meats like Poultry or pork must be cooked to a very specific minimum internal temperature for them to be safe to consume.

This risk is a risk that you take if you want to eat a raw food diet that contains meats or fish, but if they are eating a raw vegan diet, it is less of a concern.

4. Chewing

You may not know this, but digestion begins in the mouth. The first step of digestion is when you chew your food. Cooking your food makes this first step easier, and eating raw food can make it more difficult to chew, resulting in tougher digestion and more stress on the gut later on in the digestion process. If the food is in bigger pieces or not properly chewed when it reaches the gut, it can result in painful gas and bloating. Also, if you can chew your raw food thoroughly, it usually takes much more energy and effort to do so. This extra energy expenditure is especially true for meats, as they are tough and difficult to chew if they are uncooked.

5. Anti-Nutrients

There is something called an anti-nutrient that is found within some legumes, beans, and grains. Anti-nutrients are something that, when ingested, prevent the body from absorbing nutrients from the foods that contain them. However, when you cook these foods, anti-nutrients' number and effectiveness become greatly reduced, allowing your body to absorb more nutrients from the food.

6. Antioxidants

In some vegetables, their antioxidants are made more readily available to your body by cooking the vegetables, so by eating them raw, your body will be unable to extract and absorb these antioxidants. These antioxidants have been shown to reduce the risk of certain cancers and heart disease.

7. Pleasant Aroma and Appearance

Cooked food, in general, has a much more pleasant aroma and appearance than uncooked food. The first part of eating happens with your eyes and your nose. When you see and smell cooked food, your mouth begins to water, and your digestive system begins to prepare for the food to be ingested, leading to more effective digestion.

The nutrients and vitamins that a person's body can get from food are completely dependent on the body's ability to digest the food, as this is how the body gets nutrients from the food. Without proper digestion, the body is unable to extract the nutrients it needs. Thus, it is important to make an informed decision about whether to eat your food cooked or uncooked. You must consider the ease with which it can be chewed and digested and the scientific research about the availability of its nutrients and vitamins.

Further, you must examine some foods' benefits and drawbacks when cooking or eating them raw. For example, tomatoes lose some of their vitamin C content when you cook them, but their antioxidant content increases. Thus, you must make a personal decision about which you would prefer or which you need most at this stage of your life.

In some cases, some foods are better for your health, either raw or cooked. These foods and their preferred method of consumption are listed below;

- Broccoli is much healthier for the human body when consumed raw. This fact is true because there is a compound in it that has proven to be cancer-fighting, but that is found in much smaller quantities in cooked broccoli.

- Onions are beneficial for the health of your blood when consumed raw. Raw onions lead to less blood clotting but cooking them leads this benefit to be greatly reduced.

- Cabbage, when cooked for a long period, loses its beneficial enzyme for cancer prevention. Eating cabbage raw or only lightly cooked maintains much of this benefit.

- Garlic has anti-cancer benefits when it is eaten raw, but when cooked, this benefit is denatured.

- Mushrooms have been found to contain a compound that could be a carcinogen for humans. By cooking them, you are breaking down this compound and eliminating its possible harmful effects. Cooking them also releases an antioxidant that is inactive when they are raw.

- Asparagus contains many vitamins, but they are inaccessible when it is raw. The stem is so fibrous that it is difficult for the body to digest it enough to absorb these nutrients. Coking it breaks the stem down enough for the vitamins to be released and absorbed during digestion.

- Spinach contains many elements like zinc, calcium, and magnesium, but they are made much more available when cooked.

As you can see in the list above, there are some cases where you may prefer certain methods of preparation for certain foods. Keeping this in mind, a diet comprised of a mix of raw and cooked foods may be the most beneficial for most humans.

Nutrients to Include In Your Keto Diet

We have discussed briefly some of the nutrients found in certain vegetables and foods through our discussion of which foods are included in the Keto diet (with plant-based alternatives suggested). In this section, we will look at the most beneficial nutrients for your body and where/ how you can find them when following a specific diet.

Omega 3 Fatty AcidsOmega-3 Fatty Acids are needed in your diet as the body cannot make them on its own. These fatty acids are a certain type in a list of other fatty acids, but this type (Omega-3) is the most essential and beneficial for our brains and bodies in general. They have numerous effects on the brain, including reducing inflammation (which reduces the risk of Alzheimer's) and maintaining and improving mood and cognitive function, including memory. Omega-3's have these greatly beneficial effects because of how they act in the brain, making them so essential to our diets. Omega-3 Fatty Acids increase the production of new nerve cells in the brain by acting specifically on the nerve stem cells within the brain, causing new and healthy nerve cells to be generated.

Omega-3 fatty acids can be found in fish like salmon, sardines, black cod, and herring. It can also be taken as a pill-form supplement for those who do not eat fish or cannot eat enough of it. It can also be taken in the form of a fish oil supplement like krill oil.

Omega-3's are by far the most important nutrient that you need to ensure you are ingesting because of the numerous benefits of it, both in the brain and in the rest of the body. While supplements are often the last step in trying to include something in your diet, for Omega-3's, the benefits are too great to potentially miss by trying to receive all of it from your diet.

- *Sulforaphane*

Brussels Sprouts, Cabbage, Kale, Broccoli Sprouts have in common? All of these green vegetables have one thing in common- they all contain Sulforaphane. Sulforaphane is a plant chemical that is found naturally in these vegetables. Sulforaphane is an antioxidant that acts similarly to turmeric and thus has similar benefits. Sulforaphane, like turmeric, Induces Autophagy in the brain, which helps to reduce the risk of Alzheimer's, Parkinson's, and dementia, which are all neurodegenerative diseases. *Neurodegenerative* means that the cells in the brain called nerves are damaged and broken down, which leads to cognitive declines like Alzheimer's or physical decline as in Parkinson's. These vegetables can help treat these diseases by slowing their progression, as they are all diseases that come about over time. There is no cure yet, but the treatment at this stage involves delaying these diseases' progression.

Sulforaphane can be found in the vegetables mentioned above, but the strongest source is in broccoli sprouts. It can also be taken concentrated in a supplement form.

- *Calcium*

Calcium is beneficial for the healthy circulation of blood and for maintaining strong bones and teeth. Calcium can come from dairy products like milk, yogurt, and cheese. It can also be found in leafy greens like kale and broccoli, and sardines.

- *Magnesium*

Magnesium is beneficial for your diet, as it also helps you to maintain strong bones and teeth. Magnesium and calcium are most effective when ingested together, as magnesium helps in the absorption of calcium. It also helps to reduce migraines and is great for calmness and relieving anxiety. Magnesium can be found in leafy green vegetables like kale and spinach and fruits like bananas and raspberries, legumes like beans and chickpeas, vegetables like peas, cabbage, green beans, asparagus, and brussels sprouts, and fish like tuna and salmon.

- *Bioactive Compounds*

Bioactive compounds are compounds found within foods that act in the body in beneficial ways. The bioactive compounds found within berries, such as Acai Berries, Strawberries, and

Blueberries, are very beneficial for your health. The bioactive compounds in these specific types of berries work in the brain to induce Autophagy and reduce inflammation. This autophagy induction leads to the protection of brain cells, in this case, from *oxidative stress*. Oxidative stress can happen within the brain when there is an imbalance of oxygen, which can cause reduced cognitive functioning. These berries and their induction of Autophagy reduce this by keeping the balance of oxygen at a healthy level.

How to Get These Nutrients- Whole Food Sources or Supplements?

Ever since it became popular in mainstream media, the Ketogenic diet has been recommended, along with some targeted supplements to assist with aid weight loss. Below is a list of some of the most effective supplements to take in tandem with a plant-based ketogenic diet. Supplements like MCT Oil, keto protein powders, keto electrolytes, digestive enzymes, omega-3, iron, and Vitamin-D have been known to help those on a Keto diet.

While it is always better to get your nutrients, vitamins, and minerals from your whole food sources, if you are struggling to include everything you need in your diet, you can supplement to ensure you are getting all of the nutrients you need. Below you will find some of the most common supplements that people on the keto diet turn to.

Exogenous Ketones

Suppose you are proving unable to bring your carbohydrate intake to the level needed to put the body toward the nutritional ketosis environment. In that case, you may consider taking exogenous ketones as a supplement as a solution to this problem.

When tested on animal models, even when they ate according to a normal carbohydrate intake diet, these exogenous ketones proved beneficial in helping the models with problems like seizures, cancer prevention, anti-inflammation anti-anxiety. We normally see these diseases improved by Ketosis, just like we saw in this book's first few chapters.

MCT Oil

You may have heard of this oil before. MCT oil is an oil that is made up of medium-chain triglycerides, hence the name. These are fatty substances that have been shown to help people following a keto diet to add more fat to stay in a state of Ketosis. This fat type is digested more quickly than dietary fats, so it is a good way to ensure you stay in Ketosis. However, there are possible side-effects related to digestion.

Keto Protein Powders

There are protein powders made specifically for keto dieters, which contain high protein content. However, no added sugar and little-to-no carbohydrates help you maintain your muscle mass while still limiting your carb intake.

Keto Electrolytes

When you first begin eating according to a ketogenic diet, having Electrolyte depletion is quite common. This electrolyte depletion happens because of water weight loss through fat loss. It can also happen because of the lowered carbohydrate intake that accompanies the keto diet, as we have discussed. Taking electrolyte supplements, like magnesium, potassium, and sodium, can help avoid a deficiency in common electrolytes. This possible complication is also why you should ensure you are getting enough dietary sodium, as this is an electrolyte that you need. Along with this, though, you will need to ensure you are drinking enough water to avoid dehydration.

Digestive Enzymes

Because of its high-fat content, the keto diet can lead some people to have various digestive issues. By taking some form of a digestive enzyme by way of a supplement, (lipase, for example), this can help you relieve these digestive issues.

Omega-3

As you know, Omega-3 is an essential fatty acid, which means that we must consume it and that our bodies cannot create it. While we can get it in our diet, if you are eating according to a strict diet like Keto, vegan, or even vegetarian, you may have some trouble getting it. If this is the case, you should supplement it in pill form so that you can ensure your brain is functioning in tip-top shape and that your baby's brain is forming healthily as well.

Iron

This one is a little tricky, but it is worth noting. Iron should be obtained in the right amounts in your diet through whole foods. If you feel like you might be deficient in iron and have trouble getting it in the foods you eat, you can visit your doctor for advice on this topic. Iron cannot be supplemented without being referred by a doctor first, as it is something that they would like you first to try to get from your food. If this is becoming a problem, they can give you supplements to take. This deficiency is especially a concern if you are not eating much red meat, which may lead your doctor to want you to begin supplementing. Make an appointment with your doctor to find out more about this topic.

Vitamin D

Vitamin D is found in some foods that have been fortified with it, but it can be found in only a few foods in a natural sense. These include cheese, fatty fish like salmon and tuna as well as egg yolks. Another source is mushrooms that have been exposed to UV rays, so the organic ones are likely of this sort. Vitamin D can be absorbed naturally through sun exposure, so if you live in a sunny place, make sure you get our for some walks or some timer with the sun on your skin. If you live in a colder or more gloomy place, consider purchasing a lamp that mimics the sun and provides you with vitamin D in your house. On a sunny day, even if it is cold, going outside and getting sun on your face will give you vitamin D. This one is something that everyone should be conscious of, but it is especially necessary to examine if you are following a specific diet.

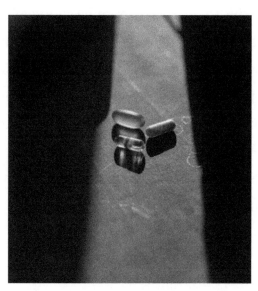

What Are Macronutrients and Micronutrients?

- **Macronutrients** are those nutrients that are comprised of other smaller nutrients. These macronutrients are carbohydrates, protein, and fat. These are the things that you will often hear about when talking about a food's content and its level of "healthiness."

- **Micronutrients** are those smaller nutrients that are the components of *Macronutrients,* such as iron or sodium. These components are found in natural food sources, and they form larger nutrients. One example of this is red meat (the macronutrient protein), which is comprised of iron (a micronutrient).

CHAPTER 4: WEIGHT LOSS

A Ketogenic diet is greatly beneficial for losing weight for people who can stick with the diet rules. Since more and more plant-based people have decided to pursue the Keto diet, we must consider plant-based alternatives to further explore Keto's role in weight loss. There are benefits to both a plant-based diet and a ketogenic diet; their benefits combine to make a very beneficial diet for your health and your waistline. We will delve into the specific ways that a Ketogenic diet can lead to rapid weight loss. First, though, we will discuss weight loss as a general concept.

Why People Over 50 Should Watch Their Weight

When it comes to the population of people over the age of 50, there are some things that they must keep in mind when it comes to weight loss. Studies show that dieting and inducing a state of Ketosis can have very beneficial effects for women and men over 50.

Since many women in this age group experience annoying and persistent belly fat, one specific research study looked at this kind of fat and how it affects women over age 50. In this study, inducing Autophagy helped women over 50 lose belly fat, leading to improvements in overall health. This weight loss also proved to lead to more satisfaction in terms of physical appearance and life satisfaction overall.

By reducing belly fat, women over 50 were able to reduce their risk of metabolic syndrome, which is especially prevalent in people in this age group. People over age 50 are at a greater risk of developing excess belly fat that is hard to remove, and approaching weight loss from this perspective made their stubborn belly fat dissipate much quicker.

How the Keto Diet Will Help With Weight Loss

The ketogenic diet helps you lose weight by combining four dietary fundamentals; hunger and satiety, water weight, fewer carbohydrates, Autophagy, and metabolism. This chapter will help you understand how these four fundamentals work together in a ketogenic diet to help you lose weight.

1. *Hunger Management*

Any time you eat mostly plant-sourced foods or foods that are closer to their natural state, they will contain high amounts of fiber and large water content, especially in the case of vegetables. This fact means that people who eat a plant-based Keto diet will feel full earlier than those who do not and will remain full for longer. This increased satiety happens because of the high fiber and the high water content, filling a person's stomach much quicker than other foods would.

Vegetables have a very low-calorie content for their size, which means that they will fill your stomach without giving you a large calorie count. Because of this, when you become full after eating a salad, for example, you will not be able to eat any more food, but you will not have ingested a large number of calories. This fullness can lead to a calorie deficit and subsequent weight loss if this type of eating is continued.

Further, studies have shown that following a ketogenic diet (high fat, low carb, moderate protein) leads to lower levels of ghrelin in the body. Ghrelin is a hormone that leads to feelings of hunger. Feeling less hungry overall and feeling fuller more quickly when you eat will lead to a decrease in calories consumed over the day and a weight reduction due to a calorie deficit.

2. Water Weight Loss

Carbohydrates hold onto a lot of water. By greatly reducing your intake of carbohydrates, you are also reducing your intake of water. By reducing the number of stored carbohydrates, you are reducing your amount of stored water. When you begin eating according to the Keto diet, your body's stored carbohydrates are used for energy quite early. At this point, you will see a reduction in weight because of the water that went along with these fat stores being used up.

3. Carbohydrate Elimination

By reducing the number of carbohydrates you intake drastically, you will be reducing the amount of sugar that you intake drastically. As we discussed previously, the more sugar you intake, the more blood sugar spikes you put your body through, which leads to an increase in stored fat. Because the blood sugar level spikes so drastically, your body releases a large amount of insulin to accommodate. It leads to fat storage, as a result, to combat the spike in blood sugar. This fat release happens, especially around the abdominal area. By switching to a diet that is low in carbohydrates and high in healthy fats, you can keep your insulin levels consistent, preventing your body from storing as much fat and encouraging your body to use fat stores for energy instead of sugars. This diet leads to a quicker metabolism, which means that the energy will be used up much quicker and more efficiently, reducing the chances of storing this energy for later. All of these things that happen as a result of reducing carbohydrate intake lead to weight loss.

4. Metabolism Changes

As we discussed earlier, Autophagy is a large part of why the Ketogenic diet is so successful in weight loss.

Metabolism is a large term that describes the breakdown of one thing to create energy. In more specific terms, it is all of the body's processes that work together to maintain life. This synchronicity happens when you eat food, and it is digested to absorb nutrients and create energy for your body to function. This synchronicity also happens on a smaller level in each cell of the body by way of Autophagy, as it aids in the breakdown of old or damaged cell components, and this breakdown creates energy for the cell.

When your body's cells are experiencing a lack of nutrition in the form of sugar, Autophagy is triggered to create more energy for the cell to use by breaking down cell parts. Along with this, the body releases hormones by the body to use the energy that it is creating in the most efficient way possible. These hormones make the body's fat stores more easily broken down and more accessible as a source of energy. Thus, the body's metabolism rate increases during these times of cellular starvation, and the body loses fat, resulting in weight loss. Therefore, the more often that your body is in a state of Ketosis, the more often this process of Autophagy will be occurring.

How the Body Loses Weight

The most basic weight loss concept is that you must put your body in a calorie deficit to lose weight. This deficit means that you must eat fewer calories than you burn, which will result in a loss of weight. The equation for this concept is below;

The number of calories that you ingest – **(minus)** The number of calories you use to survive (for example, walking, eating, breathing) – **(minus)** The extra calories burned from exercise = **(equals)** = + **(positive) or** – **(negative)**

The number that results from this equation will be either positive or negative. If the number is positive, this means that you ingested more calories than you burned. If the number is negative, this means that you burned more calories than you ingested. If the number is zero, calories ingested and calories burned are equal. If the number is zero, this indicates "breaking even" in terms of your energy. If the number is positive, you can envision it as having more energy than you could use. When this occurs, the extra energy is stored as fat in the body. If the number is negative, you used more energy than you had, which translates to weight loss, as once the energy is all used up, the fat stores will begin to be used for additional energy.

Tips for Using the Keto Diet to Lose Weight

While eating, according to a diet, promises many benefits, you must ensure that you are healthy following the diet. With this diet, in particular, it is important to ensure that you are drinking enough water. While it can be tempting to watch the pounds drop as your body loses water weight along with your decrease in carbohydrate intake, this can also leave you feeling dehydrated. Be sure to drink enough water so that you can combat the water lost through your carbohydrate stores and the lack of ingested water through the intake of carbohydrates.

Another point to note is that while you want to ensure you are at a calorie deficit to lose weight, this diet is not designed to keep you feeling hungry, and as if you are starving yourself. Instead, you should feel satisfied and full enough simply due to the food choices you are making. As I mentioned, vegetables are very low in calories for the amount of volume they occupy in your stomach, so this is a clear and effective way to avoid being left feeling hungry while still losing weight and getting all of your nutrients.

The Importance of Exercise As Part of a Diet Plan

Remember our discussion about Autophagy earlier in this book as we move onto this next section.

We discussed how Autophagy is induced by putting your body into a state of Ketosis. One other way to activate Autophagy is through exercise. Aerobic exercise has been shown through studies to increase Autophagy in the cells of the muscles, the heart, the brain, lungs, and the liver. When we do aerobic exercise, the heart and lungs work with the muscles to move the body in a specific way (like running or biking). Over time, the heart, lungs, and brain will learn to function together more efficiently, which is why exercises get easier the more you do them. Autophagy is upregulated in these specific tissues (heart, lungs, muscles) after aerobic exercise because these are the specific tissues most positively affected by aerobic exercise.

Exercise is the most efficient way to upregulate Autophagy as it happens much quicker through aerobic exercise than through starvation. The body is well-equipped to survive, and so fasting takes longer to induce Autophagy than exercise does.

When exercising, the muscles and tissues you use will experience small micro-damages, making them grow back stronger. Think of how the muscles respond after a workout in the weight room- you are sore for a few days before becoming stronger and growing bigger muscles. This soreness happens in a very similar way at a cellular level. Autophagy comes in when the cells need energy or micro-damages, clearing out the damage and encouraging new cells to take the place of the damaged ones. This process leads to growth and regeneration in the specific tissues impacted by specific exercise types. It is one of the many reasons why exercise is so beneficial for the human body.

By exercising once per day, you can feel the beneficial effects of exercise on Autophagy, and this, when compared to dieting, is much less time-consuming. For best results, combining the two will be the most effective for maintaining a healthy weight and maintaining good health, and reducing disease risk.

With exercise, it is difficult to discern which of its benefits can be attributed to an increase in Autophagy and the other bodily functions that exercise induces, like an increase in oxygen delivery to your tissues or the heart's more efficient functioning. It is being studied more and more these days, however, to understand better how much of a role Autophagy plays in recovery after exercise.

Specific Tip for People Over 50

The following tip will set you up for success as you begin following the ketogenic diet. This tip will allow you to follow your new regime without depriving yourself too strictly (as it could lead to falling off track). This tip will also help you follow your new diet plan to lose weight and prevent overeating the foods you can eat. By planning and taking care of possible roadblocks that could lead you to fall off this new plan early on, it will allow you to follow it for longer, leading to lasting weight loss.

Do Not Overeat

It is important to follow a diet plan that does not make you count calories that you do not overeat.

Since your digestive system will need to adjust to your new diet, giving it too much work to do all at once can lead to indigestion and difficulty digesting the amount of food that it has been fed, which can lead to uncomfortable side-effects for you.

There is a technique that is very helpful when it comes to preventing overeating. This technique is called "Mindful Eating." Mindful eating will come in handy, and I will begin by explaining what this technique entails.

Before we jump in, let's first learn about the basics of mindfulness. Mindfulness is most popularly achieved through the use of meditation. In our society today, psychology professionals describe meditation as a way to achieve mindfulness. Mindfulness is then described as a method of focusing one's thoughts and mind on an activity, thought, or object. This focus trains their awareness and attention. The goal of this is to help the person achieve clear-headedness and an emotionally calm and stable state. You may think that mindfulness sounds easy just by reading what it is, but it is difficult to achieve.

Mindfulness requires strong self-discipline to achieve, and simply just listening to a mindfulness podcast or going to one mindfulness class isn't going to help you become a mindful person.

The most popular reason people decide to learn meditation is to achieve mindfulness to combat mental obstacles. If you live a very fast-paced and stressful life, mindfulness and meditation can help you manage your thoughts and emotions to bring you more peace. Many doctors who specialize in mental health have begun to study and even practice meditation and mindfulness techniques to promote a healthier brain and mind. Others take the practice of meditation and mindfulness to another level and aim to reach a certain level of spirituality. When an individual can achieve mindfulness, they can increase their overall life satisfaction.

There are ways to eat that ensure you are making the most of your time eating while also getting all of the nutrients that you need when you are eating. We will talk about something called mindful eating in more detail in the next section.

By paying attention to these important areas of your life and increasing your mindfulness in them, you can begin to see areas you can improve to help you live a happier life.

Mindful eating is when you get into the moment instead of being distracted by everything going on in your mind. Mindful eating is important as these are one of those tasks that we do numerous times per day. When we do a certain task repeatedly, our bodies will naturally try to automate that action to save us energy. However, when we eat mindlessly, we don't pay attention to the way food tastes, what we're eating, and how quickly we consume it. These bad automation habits are what causes us to mistreat our body. In this section, I will teach you about mindful eating, how you can eat mindfully, and provide you with some exercises to help you eat better to improve your mindfulness.

The lack of mindful eating is something most of our population suffers from due to our lives' increased pace. We typically find ourselves eating at work in front of our computer, eating dinner in front of the TV, or even eating during the commute to work! This seemingly small problem is one of the leading factors in today's obesity and eating disorder problem. To combat this, we need to improve our ability to eat mindfully. Mindful eating incorporates mindfulness with a daily task to aid people in overcoming common problems related to digestion that many people experience with their fast-paced lives. Mindful eating is done to help people pull themselves away from incessant thinking while eating and encourages them to enjoy the food and the experience of eating. This technique is done to develop a new mindset around food. Here are a couple of points to help yourself identify when you are not practicing mindful eating.

- You often eat until you become very full and sometimes you even feel ill as a result
- You find yourself nibbling on snacks but you do not notice what you are tasting
- You aren't paying attention to your meal and you eat in places that surround you with distractions
- You are rushing through your meals
- You have trouble remembering what you ate, or even the taste and smell of the last meal you've consumed

How Can Mindful Eating Benefit You?

- *More Food Enjoyment in a Healthy Way*

If you are feeling down emotionally when you decide that it is time to eat, you may be focused on your emotional state and not tasting or enjoying the food you are eating. By practicing mindful eating, you will be present in your eating experience. This presence will help you enjoy the taste of the food and relish in a few minutes of calm to enjoy your food.

- *Better Digestion*

Being sure to eat mindfully and without distraction will help you digest better, helping you get all the nutrients you need from your food.

- *Will result in fewer food cravings*

Consciously eating will make you more aware of everything that you put into your mouth, and focusing on the experience of eating can help you to have fewer cravings and less desire to eat in between meals.

- *Prevents overeating*

Mindful eating prevents overeating because you will notice each bite you put into your mouth and be much more in tune with how you feel.

- *Improve your relationship with food*

By using mindful eating, you will not be eating as a means of making yourself feel better emotionally, but instead as nourishment for your precious body.

Practicing meditation is your first step in being able to achieve mindful eating. Allowing yourself to be mindful in your day to day life will bring new joys and satisfactions that have always been there but have not been noticed in some time, especially when it comes to eating, which you do so often.

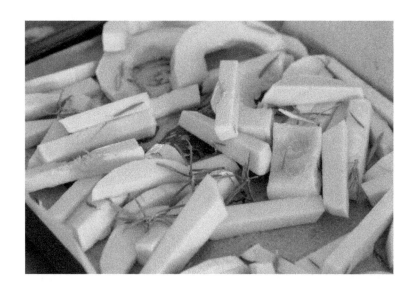

Steps Towards the Practice of Mindful Eating

If you find yourself relating to the points I outlined in the first section; you may want to practice mindful eating actively. Follow these quick exercises below to begin increasing your level of mindfulness while eating.

- **Exercise #1: Prioritize your mealtimes.**

Try to isolate a 15-minute block to sit down and enjoy your meal. Don't eat on the go or skip meals because you're 'too busy.' Ensure you are always making time to eat at least three meals per day, no matter how busy you are.

- **Exercise #2: Avoid distractions while you are eating**

You cannot focus on the food in your mouth if you are distracted. Try asking yourself how often you eat in front of the TV, in the car, or in front of the computer? Under those circumstances, eating is always mindless. Mindless eating often causes people to overeat, choose unhealthy meals, or forget to notice the taste of the food at entirely.

- **Exercise #3: Avoid rushing during meal times**

Plan a span of time in which you will eat. Make sure that your eating environment is free from distractions. Even eating with a coworker or a friend may be a distraction due to conversation.

- **Exercise #4: Always sit down to eat your meal**

When you eat, eat sitting down on a chair with your food on a table in front of you. This posture will help with digestion and help you to form a routine around eating. Try to avoid eating while standing up or walking as these create distractions. When you are physically up and about while eating, it will cause your mind to become distracted at the task at hand, as you will have to concentrate on your movement.

- **Exercise #5: Serve your meal on a plate or bowl**

If possible, serve it on your favorite plate or bowl. Avoid eating food from the packet or take out containers as it makes eating feel less formal. Doing this will help you pay more attention to your meal and its physical appearance.

- **Exercise #6: Focus on chewing completely before swallowing**

Many people find themselves swallowing too soon and end up with digestion problems. Give your stomach an easier time with digesting by breaking down the food properly before swallowing.

- **Exercise #7: Make sure only to eat until you're 80% full**

This step is a fine line. Don't eat until you are certain you are full, but eat until you feel satisfied. A lot of the time, the feeling of fullness comes 10 minutes after you finish your meal. If you find yourself feeling full while you are still eating, you probably have overeaten.

- **Exercise #8: Take your time to savor the taste of food truly**

Use all five of your senses. Before eating, take a look at your meal of its look, smell, and overall appeal. Think about how each ingredient was cooked and seasoned and how you think the dish would taste because of it. During the meal, identify the taste of all the ingredients. What is the flavor? How does the flavor change if I eat different combinations of the ingredients? How does it smell? What does the texture feel like on your tongue?

- **Exercise #9: Think about how your food makes you feel**

Does it make you happy? Pleasurable? Guilt? Regretful? Stressed out? Disappointed? Pay attention to the thoughts that the meal gives you. Does it elicit memories? Does it cause you to feel any fears? Does it remind you of certain beliefs? How does your body feel after the meal compared to before? Do you feel energetic after the meal, or does it instead cause you to experience lethargy? Is your stomach full or empty?

- **Exercise #10: Try to make meals for yourself when it is possible**

Making food for yourself is proven to be psychologically beneficial and therapeutic. Make sure you are touching, tasting, and smelling the individual ingredients.

- **Exercise #11: Make a note of the difference in good food**

This step means to make a note of your food in the following ways: This tends to be food that is fresh, seasonal, and minimally processed. Fresh and organic food tends to improve your overall mood and health. Food is our body's nourishment, and it provides the nutrition necessary for us to function optimally. Ingesting better quality food and ingredients is crucial to helping you feel better physically and psychologically.

How to Practice Mindful Eating

The key to mindful eating is to use all five of your senses. This sensual eating will bring your consciousness and state of awareness into the present moment and help you avoid distractions. To practice mindful eating, try following along with the exercise below during your next meal. Further, try to do so every meal after that. Eventually, you will be able to practice this every time you eat.

Before you take a bite of your food, notice the smells of the food you are about to eat. Notice how it looks- the colors and textures. As you put food in your mouth, feel the textures of the food on your tongue. Notice all of the flavors that you are tasting and the feeling that they bring to your mouth. Notice how it feels when you chew the food- how it feels on your teeth and your cheeks. Doing this with every bite will bring you into the moment and ensure that you are consciously eating every time that you eat. Try practicing this every time you eat.

Practicing this type of eating will help you enjoy the food and appreciate it, but it will help you to eat slowly. By taking your time with each bite and ensuring that you chew it and taste it, eating slower will naturally occur. Further, as you learned earlier in this chapter, meal planning- especially portion planning, is another way to ensure you do not overeat when you begin your new diet.

CHAPTER 5: DETERMINING YOUR PERSONAL KETO DIET PLAN

If you thought you left math class behind in high school, think again! In this chapter, we are going to look at how to calculate your daily intake!

Reminder: what are macronutrients and micronutrients?

Remember earlier in this book when we discussed Macronutrients and micronutrients? These two types of nutrients will return to this chapter. I have outlined them for you below;

- **Macronutrients** are those nutrients that are comprised of other smaller nutrients. These macronutrients are carbohydrates, protein, and fat. These are the things that you will often hear about when talking about a food's content and its level of "healthiness."

- **Micronutrients** are those smaller nutrients that are the components of *Macronutrients,* such as iron or sodium. These components are found in natural food sources, and they form larger nutrients. One example of this is red meat (the macronutrient protein), which comprises iron (a micronutrient).

What Are These Calculations Useful for?

It is important to get an idea of your amount of calories and fat and protein intake to determine if you are eating enough, too much, or just the right amount. This calculation is helpful when it comes to weight loss. Remember is an earlier chapter when we discussed weight loss and how a calorie deficit is needed to achieve weight loss? This section is where we revisit that concept. If you determine your regular daily intake, this tells you the number of calories that you would need to eat to maintain your weight exactly where it is currently. Then, to lose weight, you will reduce this number of calories slightly, and you will put yourself in a calorie deficit each day, resulting in weight loss over time. You do not need to severely restrict your calories to do this, only to have a small deficit, which will lead you to lose weight over time.

This calculation is based on age, sex, height, weight, and activity level, as all of these factors influence your body's use of calories and each macronutrient in particular.

How to Determine Your Personal Calorie Count

To begin, you will need to calculate your BMR or Basal Metabolic Rate. This calculation is an indicator of the number of calories your body needs to live simply. These "living calories" include: breathing, talking, moving, and so on, without any exercise. The bigger the person's body, the more calories they will need to maintain life. The reason that this calculation considers age is that as we get older, our amount of muscle generally decreases. Thus, we must consider this to reduce the number of calories needed to run our body's functions. Further, there is a different calculation for men than for women, as male bodies and female bodies use energy differently. You can see these equations below—plug in your own numbers to get your personal BMR.

BMR (Basal Metabolic Rate) Calculation for Men
66+ (6.2 x weight in pounds) + (12.7 x Height in inches) − (6.76 x Age) = BMR

BMR (Basal Metabolic Rate) Calculation for Women
655.1 + (4.35 x weight in pounds) + (4.7 x Height in inches) − (4.7 x Age) = BMR

The next factor contributing to the calculation of your macronutrients is to determine your TDEE or your Total Daily Energy Expenditure. This number will tell you how much energy your body uses daily, including your exercise. While BMR tells you how much energy you use if you were to just live for a day without spending any extra energy, TDEE will give you a more realistic number as it will include your level of activity.

1.2 little to none

1.375 1-3 days of light exercise

1.55 3-5 Days of moderate exercise

1.725 6-7 Days of Hard exercise

1.9 Very intense

To determine your activity level, you can include everything you do during a regular day that includes more strenuous activity than just sitting, standing, or regular walking. Depending on your job, this could be part of your activity level, such as if you are on your feet all day or lift heavy objects.

Total Daily Energy Expenditure (TDEE) Calculation for both women and men;

BMR x (your personal levels of exercise) = TDEE

This number will give you a better idea of the number of calories your body uses in a day, and we will look at how you can adjust this to determine the number of calories you should eat to lose weight shortly.

Body Fat Percentage

This step is a little difficult to determine since you need some calculation method to determine it. Your body fat percentage is a more accurate way to determine your weight than stepping on a scale since it will break down the percentage of your body weight made up of fat. This number will help you determine the amount of weight you want to lose and what a healthy amount of weight would be for your body to lose. Knowing this will also help determine how much protein you need to intake to maintain your muscles. There are multiple ways to determine your body fat percentage.

- *Skinfold Caliper*

This method is the most common method of measuring body fat percentage. This method involves taking measurements of the extra skin on your body. This tool pinches your skin and determines the amount of fat layer you have in different body areas to determine an overall percentage.

- *Measuring Tape*

You can also measure body fat percentage with a measuring tape. You would take measurements of your hips, neck, and waist and would then be able to determine your body composition, including the fat percentage. This method gives a more general idea than some of the other methods, which tend to be more accurate.

- *X-Ray Scan*

If you have access to this at your doctor's office or a clinic of some sort, you can measure your body fat percentage with this special type of X-ray called a DEXA scan. This method is the most accurate but the most difficult to get your hands on. It measures your bone density and uses this to determine your body fat percentage for you.

- *Body Fat Percentage Scale*

There is a scale that can give you more specific readings than a classic bodyweight measurement scale. This scale is called a Tanita scale. Some gyms or doctor's clinics will have these. It measures your total body weight, your fat percentage, and even your water content when you step on it. This method can give you a pretty accurate read of your body composition.

- *Visually Estimating*

If the other methods are not accessible to you, you can visually estimate your body fat percentage. This estimation would give you the most general and least specific idea and help you get an idea nonetheless. You would examine your body to determine how much fat you have versus muscle. Keep in mind that some of your body weight will include ingested water.

Lean Body Mass Calculation

Once you know your body fat percentage using one of the previously mentioned methods, you can determine your lean body mass. This calculation will use your body fat percentage and your total weight to determine your fat by weight. A second calculation will then use this to determine your lean body mass, which is essentially your body weight minus your fat mass. The calculation is below.

Body fat mass (lbs) = Total weight x body fat percentage as a decimal

Lean body mass (lbs) = Total bodyweight – fat mass in pounds

These two calculations will help you determine how much protein you need to consume to maintain your lean body mass. We will look at how to do that later on in this chapter.

Now that you know how many calories you burn daily, you can adjust this amount to put yourself in a caloric deficit, which will lead to weight loss. If you want to maintain your weight, you will eat exactly as many calories as you need to sustain your life and activity level (TDEE). If, however, you want to lose weight, this is what you will do. To begin losing weight, the recommended caloric reduction is between 10 and 20%. It is not advised to reduce your caloric intake by any more than 30%, as this can leave you without enough energy to sustain your regular activity and daily life. To get the number of calories you should eat to lose weight, you will do the following calculation;

Calorie Intake for Weight Loss = 10% reduction in TDEE
  = 0.1 x TDEE

If you were looking to reduce your calories by 20%, you would do the same equation, but substitute 0.1 for 0.2 instead. Then, you will take this number and subtract it from your TDEE. An example of this can be seen in the Sample Calculations section below.

Determine Your Personal Carbohydrate Intake

When determining your carbohydrate intake, it is important to look at your actual useable carbohydrates, equal to your total carbohydrate intake minus your fiber intake. This calculation happens because your body cannot get carbohydrates from the fiber. To determine your carbohydrate intake on a Plant-Based ketogenic diet, in particular, you will use the following equation;

$$\frac{\text{TDEE x (\% of calories)}}{4} = \text{Grams of carbohydrates per day}$$

$$\frac{\text{TDEE x (0.05)}}{4} = \text{Grams of carbohydrates, 5\% of daily calorie intake}$$

$$\frac{\text{TDEE x (0.1)}}{4} = \text{Grams of carbohydrates, 10\% of daily calorie intake}$$

For this calculation, be sure to use your TDEE that you took ten percent off of, as we calculated in the previous step, so that you are determining your carbohydrate intake based on your caloric deficit. Because the ketogenic diet includes between 5 and 10 percent carbohydrates, we will determine a range. We will do this calculation using both 0.05 and 0.1 substituted for a percentage to determine your carbohydrate range.

Determine Your Personal Protein Intake

Protein will be about 20-25% of your intake on the Keto diet. As you know now, this number will be determined by your body fat composition or your lean mass content. This fact is because the amount of protein you will eat will be largely dependent on the amount of muscle you have. This calculation is a little confusing, so read closely.

For those who are sedentary, use the following calculation;

Lean Body Mass in pounds x 0.6 grams of protein = protein intake in grams

Lean Body Mass in pounds x 0.8 grams of protein = protein intake in grams

For those who are moderately or lightly active, use the following calculation;

Lean Body Mass in pounds x 0.8 grams of protein = protein intake in grams

Lean Body Mass in pounds x 1.0 grams of protein = protein intake in grams

For those who lift weights or who want to gain muscle, use the following;

Lean Body Mass in pounds x 1.0 grams of protein = protein intake in grams

Lean Body Mass in pounds x 1.2 grams of protein = protein intake in grams

These above calculations will give you a range of protein intake in grams. If you want to determine what this is in calories, you will multiply them by 4.

Protein intake in grams x 4 = Calories from protein.

Determine Your Personal Fat Intake

On a Ketogenic diet, the majority of the calories you intake will come from fat. This section will look at our final calculation, how much fat you will need to intake, even when trying to lose weight. Fat will make up 70-80% of your total caloric intake. This calculation will be the easiest, as we already know the carbohydrate and protein intake. The fat intake will depend on the amount of protein you need, which is why these calculations are so personal to your existing body composition and your goals of gaining muscle, losing weight, or both.

100- (Protein Percentage + Carbohydrate Percentage) = Fat percentage

Example Calculations

The following calculations are a sample for a woman who is 35, weighs 143lbs, and is 5'6 in height. Her level of daily physical activity includes moderate exercise 3-5 days per week. Her body fat percentage is 26%.

BMR = 655.1 + (4.35 x 143) + (4.7 x 66 inches) – (4.7 x 35)

= 655.1 + 622.05 + 310.2 – 164.5

= 1422.85

TDEE= BMR x activity level

    = 1422.85 x 1.55

    = 2205.42 calories

Body Fat Mass = 143 x 0.26

               = 37.18 lbs

Lean Body Mass = 143lbs – 37.18 lbs

              = 105.82 lbs

Calorie Intake for Weight Loss = 10% reduction in TDEE

    = 0.1 x TDEE

    = 0.1 x 2205.42

    = 220.54 calories = 10% of your TDEE

    = TDEE- 220.54 calories

    = 2205.42 – 220.54

    = 1984.88 calories

Grams of carbohydrates, 5% of daily calorie intake = $\dfrac{\text{TDEE x } (0.05)}{4}$

$$= \dfrac{1984.88 \times 0.05}{4}$$

$$= 99.24 / 4$$

$$= 24.81$$

Grams of carbohydrates, 10% of daily calorie intake = <u>TDEE x (0.1)</u>

$$\frac{}{4}$$

$$= \frac{1984.88 \times 0.1}{4}$$

$$= 198.49 / 4$$

$$= 49.62$$

Therefore, based on our calculations, this person would be able to eat between 25 and 50 grams of carbohydrates per day.

Lean Body Mass in pounds x 0.8 grams of protein = protein intake in grams

105.82 lbs x 0.8 = 84.66 grams

84.66 grams x 4 = 338.6 calories from protein

Lean Body Mass in pounds x 1.0 grams of protein = protein intake in grams

105.82 lbs x 1.0 = 105.82 grams

105.82 grams x 4 = 423.28 calories from protein

Fat percentage = 100- (Protein Percentage + Carbohydrate Percentage)

$$= 100- (25 \text{ percent} + 10 \text{ percent})$$

$$= 100- 35$$

$$= 65\% \text{ Fat intake}$$

Fat percentage = 100- (Protein Percentage + Carbohydrate Percentage)

$$= 100- (20 \text{ percent} + 5 \text{ percent})$$

$$= 100- 25$$

$$= 75\% \text{ Fat intake}$$

The first calculation above uses the upper threshold of protein and carbohydrate intake percentage, and the second uses the lower threshold. Therefore, this woman's fat intake should come from 65-75 percent of her total calorie intake.

1984.88 x 0.65 = 1290.17 calories

$$= 65 \text{ percent of total calories}$$

Number of grams of fat = 1290.17 / 9

$$= 143.35 \text{ grams}$$

1984.88 x 0.75 = 1488.66 calories

$$= 75 \text{ percent of total calories}$$

Number of grams of fat = 1488.66 / 9

$$= 165.41 \text{ grams}$$

Therefore, this woman should be eating a total of 1985 calories per day with the following macronutrient intake;

99- 198 Calories from carbohydrates
338- 423 Calories from protein
1290- 1489 calories from fat

To achieve her desired caloric intake and avoid going over, she will need to keep track of her macronutrient intake since it is a range. Sticking to the lower end of the range will leave her below 1985, and sticking to the upper threshold will leave her somewhere around 2100 calories, so she will need to be mindful. However, this will give her flexibility in her food choices and daily meal choices, as long as these choices stay within these calculations' parameters. These calculated parameters will keep her in Ketosis and will lead her on the path to losing weight.

CHAPTER 6: WHAT HAPPENS TO THE BODY AFTER AGE 50?

This book is written specifically for those over age 50. When you reach this age group, there are different things to keep in mind than there were in your younger years. Now that you have reached this age range, you will need to take care of your health in new and different ways, and the Keto diet is one of those ways. In this chapter, we will focus on why the keto diet is so beneficial for people over age 50.

Things to Keep In Mind for People Over 50

Every person has multiple Circadian Rhythms. A Circadian Rhythm is a 24-hour cycle within the body of a living being. There are three main rhythms. These include body temperature, hormones, and sleep. Each of these rhythms has a cycle that repeats itself every 24 hours, which explains why you feel tired around the same time each night and why you may wake up automatically at the same time every morning. The same goes for hormones and temperature, but these go on without us noticing them. Your body changes its temperature and has a cycle of releasing hormones similarly as the sleep-wake cycle happens rather automatically.

When it comes to the sleep-wake cycle, it can be affected by external factors. The main factor influencing the sleep-wake cycle, or the Internal Body Clock is Sunlight and Darkness.

When there is sunlight, your body reads this as the time that it is meant to be awake, and when there is darkness, it then knows that it is time to sleep. For this reason, jet lag is such a difficult cycle to get out of, as it throws off your internal sleep-wake cycle because of the hours of lightness and darkness changing dramatically. When it is dark outside, some processes happen within your brain that tell the body it is time to wind down for sleep. It is at this time that the hormone Melatonin is released in your brain. You may have heard of melatonin before or seen it in pill-form at the drug store. The release of melatonin is what makes you feel tired in the evening around your "bedtime." Melatonin helps you to fall asleep and to stay deeply asleep throughout the night. The release of melatonin is associated with autophagy within the brain, so it is important to maintain a regular, consistent sleep-wake cycle. If your sleep-wake cycle becomes mixed up by something like shift work or inconsistent sleeping hours, it will make it difficult for the brain to produce and release adequate melatonin levels, and they may not be released at the times that you need them. This mix up is why some people choose to take melatonin as a supplement to get their sleep-wake cycle back on track by helping their brains out a little bit. It is important not to take too much melatonin in pill-form; however, as sometimes your brain could begin to rely on its supplementation, this could disturb its natural production in the brain.

Sleep Optimization

There are many ways to optimize your sleep and numerous benefits to doing so. Ensuring that you are working with your body's natural clock will ensure that you are getting adequate restful sleep, which will give you optimal brain functioning and allow your brain to perform autophagy. Autophagy in the brain, as you know, has many benefits related to disease prevention and health in general. The brain is the center of the body's functioning and controls everything we do, so keeping it healthy is very important. Optimizing your sleep allows you to have proper melatonin production, give you the best sleep quality possible and keep your sleep-wake cycle on track. Below, we will look at some ways to optimize your sleep.

- *Sunlight*

Ensuring that you are exposed to sunlight during the day, especially in the morning, will tell your brain and body that it is time to wake up and begin the day. This light signals to the brain to begin the functions that it performs during the day and stop those it does during the night. Exposing yourself to sunlight will also help show your body and brain the difference in lightness between day and night to perform its nightly functions properly.

- *Sleep-Wake Schedule*

To allow your body to perform its functions triggered by the time of day, having a consistent sleep-wake schedule is important. If your body can expect your sleep and wake times, it can perform its scheduled functions, which will make you tired at the right time and wake up at the right time. Keeping a consistent sleep-wake schedule will also help you to have maximum brain functioning throughout the day. If you surprise your body by sleeping and waking up at different times each day, you will likely wake up tired and groggy with a confused internal clock.

- *Turn Off The Phone Before Bed*

The blue light that your phone and computer give off can negatively impact your melatonin production. Exposing your eyes to blue light in the evening before bed can leave your brain and body, thinking that it is still daytime, as it cannot tell the difference between this blue light and sunlight. Because of this, it will think it is still daytime. It will not produce melatonin when it needs to, leading you to experience difficulty falling asleep and difficulty staying asleep throughout the night.

Besides your phone and laptop, your house lights, if they are LED, can give off blue light; your television and your desktop computer do as well. When it becomes dark outside, turn off any LED lights in your house or change your lightbulbs to the soft yellow kind, do activities that do not involve screens like reading or listening to podcasts, or take a relaxing shower. If you must use electronic devices, you can download applications that will cut the blue light on your computer or your phone screen after sunset, helping your body know that it is nighttime. You can also wear blue light blocking glasses to avoid exposing your eyes to this type of light after sunset. These would be especially beneficial around daylight savings time when the sun sets rather early. Further to this point is what you are using your phone or laptop for right before bed. If you are watching or reading stimulating things that are making your heart race or your mind run, this will make it difficult for you to relax enough to fall asleep. Your brain may also continue processing these things into the night, which can lead to nightmares and interrupted sleep.

- *Avoid Eating Before Bed*

When you eat right before bed, it can be difficult to fall asleep as your digestive system will begin running, and this will give you a jolt of energy when you want to be winding down instead. Sitting up or standing during digestion also helps your body digest properly, and lying down right after eating can cause indigestion. This indigestion can interrupt your sleep, as well. It is recommended to avoid eating less than three hours before bed to give your body ample time to digest and relax again.

- *Caffeine*

Whether you are feeling tired or not, sometimes caffeine in the afternoon can make your sleep quality diminished and can make for a night of restless sleep. Try to avoid having caffeine after 3 pm so that you can let your body perform its natural nightly functions without them being interrupted by the presence of pesky caffeine molecules.

- *Complete Darkness*

Sleeping in complete darkness is beneficial for your brain as it allows your body to do all of its normal nightly functions without being confused by the presence of light. These nightly functions include generating new neurons in the brain, repairing muscles from exercise, and generally repairing and resting. If there are lights in the room or lights coming in through the window, the body and brain may become confused about whether it is getting close to sunrise and if it should begin to prepare to wake you. Sleeping in complete darkness avoids this. To do this, make sure you have blackout curtains or wear an eye mask to sleep and keep your phone turned off. If you need an alarm clock, make sure its display has orange or red light instead of blue.

- *Stress Levels*

Going to bed with high-stress levels will make it hard for your brain to calm down and enter a state of dormancy. Before bed, avoid stressful conversations and stress-inducing activities like films or tv shows that could cause you to stress or work activities like checking your emails. Take time before bed to relax and take your mind off stressful thoughts and activities to ensure you get the most restful sleep possible.

- *Alcohol*

Alcohol before bed can make it so that your brain cannot get to the deeper parts of sleep. This effect can make for a less restful sleep where autophagy is not induced as well as it should be, and neurogenesis (the building of new cells in the brain) is not accomplished to the same level that it otherwise would. This lack of deep sleep can cause you to feel tired and foggy in the morning.

- *Electromagnetic Fields*

Our phones and laptops, and other electronics are constantly giving off electromagnetic fields to stay connected to WIFI, cellular networks, and GPS. These electromagnetic fields are not something that we can see, but they can impact us without our knowledge.

In our bodies, there are constantly small electrical impulses firing, especially in the brain. In this way, different areas of our body communicate with each other to produce thoughts, movements, and automatic functions like breathing or swallowing. Because these impulses use low levels of electricity, our electronic devices' electromagnetic fields can impact the regular functioning of the electric impulses in our brain and body. In time, exposure to these, especially while sleeping, could impact the healing and generation of new cells in the brain due to insomnia or disrupted sleep. This factor's full impact is difficult to determine at this stage as it is a relatively new issue that is still being studied to be better understood.

To combat this, you should switch off your phone and laptop completely during the night, as well as your WIFI signal within your house. If you are unable to completely shut off your WIFI connection, ensure that other devices connected to it are removed from your bedroom, and those in your bedroom are switched off completely.

Optimizing Autophagy

As you can see, there are many different ways to optimize autophagy. The way or ways that you choose will be highly dependent on you as an individual. You may want to approach this by trying one and being open to changing methods if it does not work as well as you would like. You may want to try a combination of methods to get the best results. The key is to be flexible and be open to change, as nobody knows how their body will react to changes in diet and exercise.

How the Body Changes After 50

- *Insulin Sensitivity*

Remember in the previous section when we discussed **Circadian Rhythms**? We will revisit this concept once again here. It has been shown that there is a circadian rhythm of metabolism (the body's use of chemical processes to create energy) that is closely linked to the circadian rhythm of the sleep and wake cycle.

The circadian metabolic rhythm is so closely linked to the sleep-wake cycle that the quality of sleep that you get can impact the body's ability to use insulin effectively. Insulin is what regulates blood sugar by responding to sugar levels in the blood and opening or closing channels through which sugar molecules travel into and out of cells.

There are certain times within this circadian rhythm of metabolism where the body can better use insulin to regulate blood sugar and energy levels than at other times. When following a specific diet plan, you want to be aware of this cycle (circadian rhythm) and eat according to your body's ability to use insulin most effectively.

Because of the cycle of insulin sensitivity, eating according to the keto diet is beneficial for men and women over age 50. It is greatly beneficial for people over age 50 to eat a breakfast containing low to no carbohydrates. The reason for this is so that your blood sugar levels do not spike too high too quickly. Because of the lack of food that has been ingested during your time spent sleeping, your blood sugar levels will begin to accommodate this lack of food. If you suddenly feed your body a meal with high carbohydrate content, this can shock the body's insulin system. This shock to the insulin system can cause the body to suddenly work on overdrive to quickly accommodate and regulate the spike in blood sugar that the body has just experienced. If you are over 50, your body will begin to grow weaker and tired if this happens every day. For this reason, following the Keto diet will help you to keep your metabolism and your insulin system working accurately for the rest of your life.

- *Menopause*

Women over age 50 who follow the keto diet have led to the release of hormones that, in turn, lead to the release of bone minerals such as phosphate and calcium, and the release of these bone minerals leads to an increase in bone density and strength. This increase in bone minerals is especially beneficial in women over 50, as the risk of developing osteoporosis is very high in this age range. For this reason, inducing autophagy in the body by following the keto diet leads to a reduction in the risk of developing osteoporosis in women over 50. Studies show that if women follow the keto diet after age 50, they can begin to see improvements in bone density if they are already diagnosed with osteoporosis.

When it comes to menopause, many things in the body may feel like they are out of the woman's control. Menopause can lead to weight gain, depression, anxiety, an increase in their risk of heart disease, among other potential issues. Menopause can also lead to changes in hormone production and the metabolism of women experiencing menopause and a reduction in the body's sensitivity to insulin.

Because of these side effects of menopause, the keto diet is tested and proven to reduce those side effects. Further, the keto diet has shown to be useful in improving the side effects if they are already present. The keto diet has proven to be a good choice for improving the symptoms of menopause, such as the pesky weight gain that many women experiences, reducing the risk of heart disease, reducing depression, and improved cognitive functioning.

Therefore, not only can the keto diet improve the way you feel about your body and yourself/ your life in general during this time of transition, but it can also make you live a longer and healthier life.

CHAPTER 7: PUTTING THIS DIET INTO PRACTICE

One of the most daunting tasks of following a ketogenic diet is how to shop for it properly. If you are an adult, you likely have done numerous grocery shops and have gotten into a habit and routine of getting certain items every time. This habit is going to change when you take on a new diet. This chapter will teach you how to approach the grocery store and choose the right items to have a successful ketogenic diet. Let's jump right in.

Sample Shopping List

Macadamia nuts

Full-fat Greek yogurt (plain)

Eggs

Coconut oil

Extra virgin olive oil

tuna

Salmon

Avocados

Coconut milk (full fat)

Grass-fed steak

Grass-fed poultry

Spinach

Mushrooms

Feta cheese

Eggs

Coffee

Heavy cream

Salmon

Broccoli

Garlic

Onion

No sugar added

Caesar dressing

Unsweetened yogurt

Romaine lettuce

Boneless-skinless

Chicken breast

Bacon

Parmesan cheese

Extra virgin olive oil

Avocado

Turkey breast

Sour cream (full fat)

Pumpkin seeds

Grape tomatoes

Blue cheese dressing (natural)

Grass-fed ground beef

Low carb, no sugar added tomato sauce

zucchini

shirataki noodles (carb-free noodles)

pickles

cauliflower

broccoli

almonds

walnuts

eggplant

yellow squash

coconut milk (full fat)

sausage

cream cheese

cucumber

rotisserie chicken

almond butter, no sugar added

sausage links

butter

spaghetti squash

How to Plan Your Week

Planning each of your meals will make it much easier for you to reach for something nutritious and delicious when you get home from work or when you wake up tired in the morning and need to pack something for your lunch.

You can plan your meals out a week in advance, two weeks, or even a month if you wish. You can post this up on your fridge, and each day you will know just what you have ready to go in your fridge, with no thinking required. When you do this, you will be able to step up to your fridge at dinner time and choose something that you want to eat and that you know you will provide your body with the nutrients it needs. You can heat it in the oven and then begin to eat mindfully at the table. By doing this preparation and planning for yourself in advance, you will allow yourself to eat good healthy food and the right proportion of food. Since you will have already planned out your meals and their size, you are taking care of much of the thinking involved, which leaves space for you to practice mindful eating, as we discussed.

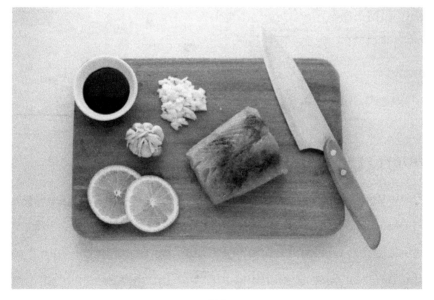

SAMPLE WEEKLY PLAN

Day 1

Breakfast:

Spinach, mushroom, and feta omelet with keto coffee (coffee with added fat such as MCT oil, butter, or bone broth protein). "This breakfast is a good source of protein and healthy fats that will keep you feeling full to curb midmorning cravings,"

Lunch:

Oven-baked salmon with broccoli. "This lunch features salmon, which is high in heart-healthy fats, as well as broccoli, which is low in carbs but high in fiber," says Dr. Axe.

Dinner:

A Chicken Caesar salad

- Chicken breast and romaine lettuce, parmesan, and some bacon.

A chicken Caesar salad is a great go-to as it is full of protein and will be just as filling as you need at dinner; this is the perfect meal to finish off your day with!

You can also add some olive oil to your dressing to pump up the fat content, as well as plenty of cheese of any type you wish.

Bonus: Snack

Bacon, Lettuce, Tomato rolls using turkey and avocado.

The BLT is a classic, and by adding turkey and avocado too, it is full of protein, fat and is virtually carb-free, perfect for your new plant-based keto diet.

If you are feeling hungry during the day in response to a lack of carbohydrates, practice eating snacks like this one so that you stay on track and fill your stomach with delicious nutrients like these.

Day 2

Breakfast:

You can use unsweetened yogurt made with whole milk and add a mix of full-fat sour cream, some berries such as strawberries, raspberries, and some seeds like flax seeds, chia seeds, and nuts like sliced almonds and walnuts. When preparing this breakfast, be sure to be mindful of your carbohydrates and portion size, counting your macros the whole time. This counting is important because, for example, all yogurt contains lactose, which is technically counted as a carbohydrate. Pair this parfait with a protein containing no carbohydrates, such as two eggs, which will help you get all of your macros in the right amounts.

Lunch:

You can eat a healthy lunch-time salad with avocado, nitrate-free, sugar-free bacon, cheese, grape tomatoes, and a variety of nuts and seeds like spicy pumpkin seeds. Add a sugar-free, low-carb, high-fat ketogenic, and plant-based salad dressing on tops, such as ranch or blue cheese dressing, or make your own with olive oil and garlic.

Dinner:

Grass-fed ground beef cooked with onions and a homemade low-carb, no sugar added tomato sauce and served alongside some grilled zucchini or eggplant, or with carb-free shirataki noodles.

If you need to get your fat intake higher in this meal, if you have not hit your macros for the day, you can sauté your zucchini in olive oil instead of grilling it, or add some extra olive oil infused with garlic directly into your sauce."

Day 3

Breakfast:

A no sugar added full-fat Greek yogurt bowl with seeds, nuts, and berries.

Coffee with 2 Tbsp Heavy Cream or half and a half

Lunch:

Make yourself a Keto lunch box that includes the following: sliced grilled chicken, organic, nitrate-free, sugar-free lunch meat such as turkey, any type of cheese cubes that you wish, pickles, a hard-boiled egg, raw tomatoes, raw vegetables such as cauliflower, carrots, radishes, or broccoli, nuts for protein and fat such as walnuts, or almonds, homemade guacamole (avocado, onion, garlic, jalapeno), and no sugar added ranch dressing.

Dinner:

Grilled chicken with a side of grilled eggplant and grilled zucchini and cherry tomatoes sautéed in extra virgin olive oil with garlic. By incorporating extra fats with oils or sauces helps to get your fat intake high. This same result can also be achieved by including coconut cream or heavy cream to keep you on track with your fat intake requirement.

Day 4

Breakfast:

Homemade Sausage & Spinach Frittata, including any vegetables you wish, such as bell peppers, onion, mushrooms, etc.

Coffee with 2 Tbsp Heavy Cream or half and a half

Lunch:

Cream cheese with cucumber slices for dipping.

(Cucumber is a low-carb and high-water content vegetable that is versatile and great for a plant-based keto diet)

Hard-boiled egg

Keto-friendly meatballs

Day 5

Breakfast:

1/2 cup Ketogenic Egg Salad with Romaine Lettuce Wraps and two slices of cooked bacon, diced.

Lunch:

Homemade guacamole (avocado, onion, garlic, jalapeno, lime juice) with raw zucchini slices for dipping.

Hard-boiled egg

Tuna

Dinner:

Approximately 6 oz of a Rotisserie Chicken

3/4 cup cauliflower gratin

As well as 2 cups chopped romaine lettuce drizzled with 2 Tbsp Caesar Salad Dressing (sugar-free)

Day 6

Breakfast:

Coffee with 2 Tbsp Heavy Cream or half and a half

Five sticks of celery dipped in 2 Tbsp of peanut or Almond Butter

Lunch:

2 cups chopped romaine lettuce with 2 Tbsp Caesar Salad Dressing (sugar-free) to make a small salad

1 cup chopped chicken (can use the chicken from the night before)

Dinner:

One Italian sausage (230 calories, 18g fat, 1g net carbs, 13g protein) with,

1 cup of cooked or raw broccoli (55 calories, 0g fat, 6g net carbs, 4g protein)

1 Tbsp butter that can be added to the broccoli for taste

2 Tbsp grated parmesan cheese that can also be added to the broccoli

Day 7

Breakfast:

2 Keto pancakes, as seen in the recipe chapter above

2 slices of bacon

Black Coffee with 2 Tbsp Heavy Cream or half and a half (heavy cream preferred)

Lunch:

1/2 cup Cauliflower "Pasta" Salad

Feta and Sundried Tomato Meatballs

2 cups raw baby spinach

Spinach can be included in the meatballs or eaten separately

Dinner:

1 1/2 cups Spicy Spaghetti Squash Casserole

Two cups of baby spinach, raw or cooked with 1 Tbsp ranch dressing (sugar-free), drizzled

MORE TIPS FOR SUCCESS

- *Enter The Store With A List*

The first thing you need to keep in mind when grocery shopping for a new diet is entering the grocery store with a list. By doing this, you will give yourself a guide, which will prevent you from picking up whatever you crave or whatever you feel like eating at that moment. IF you treat it like a treasure hunt, you will be able to cross things off of the list one at a time without venturing to the parts of the grocery store that you do not need to go in, and that will simply prove to be a challenge for you to avoid.

- *Choose Meat And Vegetables That You Love*

Since the only things that you need to stick to low-carbohydrate foods and meals, you can allow yourself some room for creativity within your shopping experience. If you prefer broccoli over tomatoes, buy broccoli and find new and fun recipes to use broccoli. If you don't enjoy eggplant, you don't have to eat eggplant at all. By giving yourself some creative freedom within your diet's parameters, you can let yourself feel a sense of choice and control over what you eat. This sense of control will help you stick to the diet and avoid feelings of an uncontrolled life, which can lead you to abandon the diet quite quickly.

- *Shop Temptation Free*

Since a ketogenic diet is high in fat and proteins, stick to your grocery store's butcher and meat areas. Avoid the middle aisles, where it is full of carbohydrates and sugars. If you are eating plant-based, you will be spending most of your time in the grocery store around the outer perimeter. This location is where the whole, plant-based foods are located. By doing this, and entering with a list, as I mentioned, you will be able to avoid the middle aisles where the processed and high-carb, high-sugar foods are all kept. This strategy will keep you away from temptations and away from foods that you will not eat on this diet.

- *Do Not Shop When You Are Hungry*

One of the biggest things that I mention to everyone when beginning the keto diet is to shop when you are hungry. This mood will make you reach for anything and everything that you see. By entering the grocery store when you are full or when you have just eaten, you will be able to stick to your list and avoid falling prey to temptations. Make sure you've had a satisfying meal before heading to the grocery store to avoid temptation buys.

SAMPLE RECIPES

CREAMY ZUCCHINI NOODLE PASTA (VEGAN, VEGETARIAN)

NUTRITIONAL INFORMATION:

One serving- half of recipe

Calories: 362

Carbohydrates: 16g

Fiber: 9.1g

Fat: 6.3g

Protein: 4.6g

10 mins: Preparation time

5 mins: Cook time

15 mins: Total

INGREDIENTS:

Water- if and as you need it

Lemon juice- 1 tablespoon

Zucchini- 3, cut to strips of ¼ inch width

Garlic- 1 clove

Avocado-1

Fresh basil- ½ cup

Salt and pepper for tasting

Olive oil- 2 tablespoons

INSTRUCTIONS:

For you to make this sauce- combine.

1. By putting the following ingredients into a food processor, blend the mixture until it becomes smooth: the avocado, basil leaves, garlic, and lemon juice and

2. Next, add the extra virgin olive oil and blend again until incorporated.

3. Add some water, 1 Tablespoon at a time, just until the sauce becomes fluid but yet still thick in its consistency.

4. Season this sauce with pepper and salt, to taste.

5. If you have never made them before, make the Zucchini Noodles before: use a spiral machine or slice them into thin, noodle-shaped strips.

6. Once you have made your noodles, sauté them in a small amount of olive oil on medium to medium-high temperature until they become softer and a brighter green hue. This change will usually take about 4 minutes.

7. Drain out the extra water from the pan, and you are ready to serve.

8. **To Serve:** Toss your zucchini noodles in the sauce you made and add some parmesan cheese to the top.

9. (you will likely have some sauce for leftovers, depending on how many macros you are looking to take in).

CAPRESE SALAD WITH BEETS AND AVOCADO (VEGETARIAN)

NUTRITIONAL INFORMATION:

Serving size (1/2 recipe)

Calories: 444

Total Carbohydrates: 5g

Fiber: 1g

Net Carbohydrates: 4g

Fat: 38g

Protein: 22g

INGREDIENTS:

Unsalted almonds, raw and chopped - ¼ cup

Avocado, sliced- 1 whole

Preservative-free, sugar-free Dijon mustard- ½ teaspoon

Fresh basil, thinly sliced- to garnish

Minced shallots- 1 tablespoon

Soft, fresh cheese of choice, sliced- 1 cup.

Beet- 1 small

Sea salt- ¼ teaspoon

Balsamic vinegar- 2 tablespoons

Extra virgin olive oil- 1 tablespoon

Freshly ground black pepper- as much as desired.

INSTRUCTIONS:

1. Preheat the oven to 400°F. Wrap the beet in foil. Roast until tender when pierced with a fork, about 1 hour. When the beet is cool enough to handle, peel it, and cut it into about eight slices.

2. Meanwhile, in a small bowl, whisk together the vinegar, shallots, oil, mustard, ⅛ teaspoon salt, and ⅛ teaspoon pepper.

3. Arrange the beet, cheese, and avocado slices on two plates and sprinkle with nuts and basil. Sprinkle evenly with the remaining salt and pepper, and drizzle evenly with the vinaigrette.

AVOCADO EGG BOWLS (VEGETARIAN)

NUTRITIONAL INFORMATION:

Serving size 130g (One half of recipe)

Calories 215

Fat 18g

Carbohydrates 8g

Fiber 2.6g

Calories from fat 163

Protein 9g

INGREDIENTS:

Coconut oil- 1 Teaspoon

Organic, free-range eggs-2

Salt and pepper- to sprinkle

Large & ripe avocado- 1

FOR GARNISHING:

Chopped walnuts, as many as you like

Balsamic Pearls

Fresh thyme

INSTRUCTIONS:

1. Slice your avocado in two, then take out the pit and remove enough of the inside so that there is enough space inside to accommodate an entire egg.

2. Cut off a little bit of the bottom of the avocado so that the avocado will sit upright as you place it on a stable surface.

3. Open your eggs and put each of the yolks in a separate bowl or container. Place the egg whites in the same small bowl. Sprinkle some pepper and salt to the whites; according to your taste, then mix them well.

4. Melt the coconut oil in a pan that has a lid that fits and put it on med-high.

5. Put in the avocado boats, with the meaty side down on the pan, the skin side up, and saute them for approx— 35 seconds, or when they become darker in color.

6. Turn them over, then add to the spaces inside, almost filling the inside with the eggs' whites.

7. Then, reduce the temperature and place the lid. Let them sit covered for approximately 16 to 20 minutes until the whites are just about fully cooked.

8. Gently add one yolk onto each of the avocados and keep cooking them for 4 to 5 minutes, just until they get to the point of cook you want them at.

9. Move the avocados to a dish and add toppings to each of them using the walnuts, the balsamic pearls, or/and thyme.

FRESH GREEN BEANS WITH BACON AND MUSHROOMS

NUTRITIONAL INFORMATION:

Serving: 1 Serving (1/6 of Recipe)

Calories: 94kcal

Carbohydrates: 9g

Protein: 5g

Fat: 5g

Saturated Fat: 2g

Fiber: 3g

Sugar: 4g

15 minutes: Prep Time

20 minutes: Cook Time

35 minutes: Total Time

Servings: 6 Servings

INGREDIENTS:

1 pound thin green beans trimmed

Three strips bacon

One large shallot minced

12 ounces mushrooms thinly sliced

One teaspoon olive oil

Three tablespoons parsley minced

One tablespoon minced fresh thyme leaves

One tablespoon minced fresh sage

1/4 teaspoon kosher salt

1/4 teaspoon freshly ground black pepper

INSTRUCTIONS:

1. Bring a large saucepan of salted water to a boil. Add the beans and cook until tender-crisp, about 2 minutes. Drain and immediately transfer the beans to a bowl of ice water to stop the cooking.

2. Drain the beans again and set aside.

3. Place the strips of bacon in a large skillet set over medium heat. Cook until the bacon is crisp. Transfer to a paper towel, then crumble the bacon and set aside.

4. Discard all but one teaspoon of the bacon fat. Add the olive oil to the bacon fat in the skillet, and turn to medium-high heat. Add the shallots and mushrooms, and cook until tender, 2 to 3 minutes.

5. Add the green beans and cook for 1 to 2 minutes, stirring frequently.

6. Add the parsley, thyme, sage, salt, and pepper, and stir to combine. Cook for an additional minute, then add the bacon.

7. Serve hot or at room temperature.

NO-BAKE CHOCOLATE PEANUT BUTTER KETOGENIC PROTEIN BARS (VEGAN)

NUTRITIONAL INFORMATION:

1 SERVING= 1 BAR

Calories: 210

Calories from fat: 124

Fat 13g

Carbohydrates: 13g

Fiber: 3g

Net Carbohydrates: 10g

Protein: 8.6g

Prep Time 10 minutes

Cook Time 30 minutes

Total Time 40 minutes

Servings 10 bars

Calories 210 kcal

INGREDIENTS:

Natural creamy peanut butter (just peanuts + salt)- ¾ cup

Organic, no sugar added Honey- ¼ cup

Melted coconut oil- 1 tablespoon

Vanilla- 1 teaspoon

Ground flaxseed meal- 1/3 cup

Plant-based protein powder- ½ cup

85% dark chocolate- 2.5 ounces

Coarse sea salt- for topping at the end

INSTRUCTIONS:

1. In a medium bowl, mix together peanut butter, honey, coconut oil, and vanilla until smooth. Add in ground flaxseed meal and protein powder of choice. Use a spoon to mix together until you can't anymore, then use clean hands to help work together. The batter should be similar to cookie dough.

2. Press into an 8x4 inch pan lined with parchment paper.

3. Make the chocolate layer by adding 2.5 ounces of dark chocolate to a small saucepan and melting until completely smooth. Pour the melted chocolate over the peanut butter layer and tilt the pan so that the chocolate covers the peanut butter layer entirely.

4. Place in the fridge for 30 minutes-1 hour before slicing into 10 bars or squares (either work, but I love squares the most)—store covered in the fridge until ready to eat. Bars will keep for up to two weeks.

CONCLUSION

It is important to remember that weight loss, a change of mind, or a change in rooted behaviors do not happen in one day or even in one week. The key to making any sort of change that will last in your life is consistency. You must be consistent in your meal planning practice, your diet, your change of behaviors, and every component of your new lifestyle to see changes. If, for some reason, you slip up, remind yourself that you are not a failure and continue where you left off. This reminder is how you maintain consistency and make changes in your life. Below are a few more tips for success that I want to leave you with.

How to Stay On Track

When it comes to making any sort of a change in life, the approach you take will make or break your success. If you choose an approach that doesn't work well with your specific personality, the likelihood of relapse will be extremely high. In this section, we will discuss the drawbacks of approaching change with an aggressive and rigid approach and the benefits of using positive reinforcement instead.

Taking an approach focused on perfection leaves you feeling down on yourself and like a failure most of the time. Because this causes you to notice that you are not perfect instead of focusing on the good parts, the progress you have made will always make you feel like you are not doing enough or have not made enough progress. Since you will never achieve perfection as this is impossible for anyone, you will never feel satisfaction or allow yourself to celebrate your achievements. You must recognize that this will be something difficult, but that you will do it anyway. If you force yourself into change like a drill sergeant and with an aggressive mindset, you will end up beating yourself up every day for something. Forcing yourself will not lead to a long-lasting change, as you will eventually become fed up with all of the rules you have placed on yourself, and you will just want to abandon the entire mission. If you approach the change with rigidity, you will not allow yourself time to look back on your achievements and celebrate yourself, to have a tasty meal that is good for your soul every once in a while, and you may fall off of your plan in a more extreme way than you were before. You may end up having a week-long binge and falling into worse habits than you had before.

It is quite difficult to avoid this when you are trying to make a change by using deprivation. It is quite rare that a person, no matter how strong their willpower, will be able to deprive themselves of something without easing off of it completely. A sudden and strict deprivation is not natural to our brains and will leave us feeling confused and frustrated.

What to Do If You Slip Up

If you are not feeling on top of your game one day or one week, recognizing and responding to this is much more effective than putting your nose to the grindstone every day and becoming burnt out, tired, and left without any more willpower. To continue on the long and difficult journey that a lifestyle change involves, you must give yourself a break now and then. Think of this like running a marathon, where you will need to go about it slowly and purposefully with a strategy in mind. If you ran into a marathon full-speed and refused to slow down or look back at all, you would lose energy, stamina, and motivation in quite a short amount of time and turn back or run off the side of the road feeling defeated and as you failed. Looking at this example, you can see that this person did not fail; they just approached the marathon with the wrong strategy. You can also see that they would have been completely capable of finishing that marathon if they had taken their time, followed a plan, and slowed down every once in a while to regain their strength. Even if they walked the marathon slowly for hours and hours, they would eventually make it over that finish line. They would probably also do so feeling proud, accomplished, and like a new person. This perspective is how we want to view this journey or any journey of self-improvement. Even if you take only one tiny step each day, you are taking a step toward your goal, and that is the important part. Even if a person has all the best intentions and the most well-made plans, sometimes they will fall short when practicing self-discipline. Avoiding failure altogether is impossible, and we should not build a mindset around that. Everyone will have their ups and downs, their successes, and their failures. The key to overcoming the failures that you will face is simply to keep moving forward. If you stumble on your journey of self-discipline, instead of giving up altogether, acknowledge what caused it, learn from it, and then move on. Don't let yourself get caught up in frustration, anger, or guilt because these emotions are the ones that will de-motivate you and get in the way of your future progress. Learn from the mistakes you have made and be comfortable with forgiving yourself. Once you have done that, you can get your head back in the game and start where you left off.

Next Steps

As you take all of this information forth with you, it may seem overwhelming to begin applying this into your own life. Remember, life is a process, and you do not need to expect perfection from yourself. By taking steps to read this book, you are already on your way to changing your life. IF you fall off of the diet and you need inspiration, come back to the first chapters of this book and remind yourself why you wanted to begin it in the first place. After reading this book, the next steps are to begin your calculations for your intake if you have not done that yet. Next, read through the multitude of recipes in this book and determine which ones you want to try first. Go ahead and make yourself a meal plan or use the 7-day meal plan in the last chapter of this book. Make yourself a grocery list or use the one provided and rid your house of any temptation foods if you can- refined carbohydrates and sugars will be the worst culprits. Then, you will have no choice but to follow the diet when you are cooking at home, and by having your weekly meals planned out for you already, you are setting yourself up for success. Ever since it began to become popular in mainstream media, the Ketogenic diet has been recommended, along with some targeted supplements to assist with aid weight loss. Below is a list of some of the most effective supplements to take in tandem with a plant-based ketogenic diet. Supplements like MCT Oil, keto protein powders, keto electrolytes, digestive enzymes, omega-3, iron, and Vitamin-D has been known to help those on a Keto diet.

I hope that through reading this book, you have developed a deeper knowledge of how you can begin to change your life in much deeper ways than just losing weight, but by also acknowledging and tackling problems before they arise. I wish you luck in your journey, and I hope that you continue to pursue lasting change.

9 798566 896496